LYN MARSHALL'S
EVERYDAY YOGA

LYN MARSHALL'S

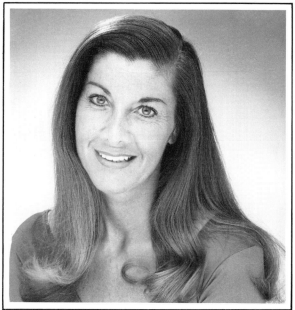

EVERYDAY
YOGA

BBC BOOKS

This book accompanies the BBC Television
series *Lyn Marshall's Everyday Yoga*

The series is presented by Lyn Marshall
and produced by Peter Ramsden

The photographs for the book are by Chris Ridley

Published to accompany a series
of programmes prepared in consultation with the
BBC Continuing Education Advisory Council

©Lyn Marshall 1982
First published 1982
Reprinted 1983, 1986
Reissued 1988
Published by BBC Books, a division of BBC Enterprises Limited,
Woodlands, 80 Wood Lane, London W12 0TT

This book is typeset in Monophoto Gill Sans
Printed in England by Jolly & Barber Ltd, Rugby

ISBN 0 563 21372 8

CONTENTS

THE AUTHOR

Lyn Marshall accidentally discovered Yoga while working as a professional dancer and model, and developed her own style of Yoga by turning the classical positions into slow, stretching Yoga movements.

Having trained as a dancer from the age of four, Lyn was well aware of how hard and unpleasant it can be to get and keep the body in shape, and was therefore not prepared for the amazing results she saw in herself when she started to do these slow gentle Yoga stretches regularly. Other people around Lyn also noticed these remarkable changes and wondered how anything so pleasant and easy to do could be so beneficial. They persuaded her to teach them her style of Yoga and before long, the demand was such that Lyn was teaching full time.

Lyn has now been teaching her special style of Yoga for thirteen years and has an ever widening circle of students, both in her London classes and through television and in print.

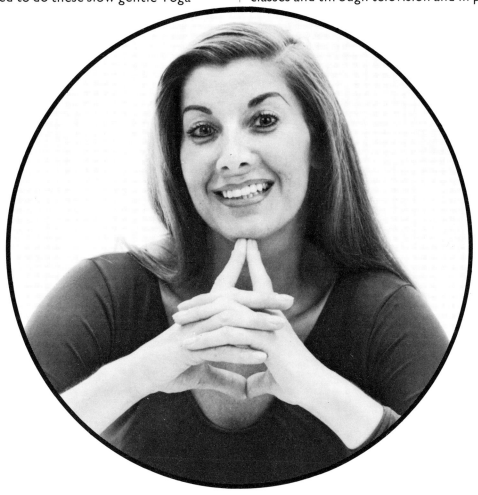

INTRODUCTION

Since I became involved in Yoga thirteen years ago, I have wanted to write a book that showed not only how wonderfully simple and easy this style of Yoga is to do, but also how to link the various movements in the right order so that the book automatically forms a complete Yoga routine you can do in your own home.

I am delighted to say that, with this book, I have finally achieved my aim and have specially selected some basic Yoga movements for your routine, that are not only easy, simple and enjoyable to do, but when linked in this way, form a comprehensive sequence that moves and improves virtually every part of you.

You can start immediately whether you are a complete beginner or not, and no matter what your age, sex or occupation, my *Everyday Yoga* routine is designed for *you*. That means you don't have to worry about which movements you ought to do for which part of your body, or which of the movements go together and which don't. I have done it all for you, and you simply have to do the movements in the order shown in the book. As you will see, you begin by relaxing in a special position, and then the movements flow on naturally, one from the other, until you come to that same relaxation position again at the end of the routine.

I have called this book *Everyday Yoga* and, indeed, if you are lucky enough to have the time, you should practise daily. However if, like many people, your time is more limited, two or three times a week is fine, or even once a week. The benefits of this style of Yoga are so great that, compared to conventional exercise, far less practice is actually needed. As long as the routine is performed slowly and smoothly as instructed, without rushing through it or trying to go that little bit further, you will begin to feel good from your very first session, and may subsequently find yourself making time to do the routine more often.

You need no special equipment to do the routine, just you, your copy of *Everyday Yoga* and the space in which to do it. So start today, and see how easy it is to firm, stretch, condition and relax every part of you without exertion or strain.

I hope you enjoy your *Everyday Yoga* routine and that like countless others it will become an essential part of a richer, healthier and happier life for you.

Lyn Marshall

I want to tell you a little about this style of Yoga and its benefits, how something as pleasurable, easy and effortless can have such a dramatic effect on your mental, physical and emotional health and how this style of Yoga differs from some of the other styles that you may have seen or heard about. However, if you are impatient to begin practising the routine, turn to the Practice Section on page 19, making sure that you read through it before you actually start.

WHAT IS THIS KIND OF YOGA AND HOW DOES IT WORK?

For a start, I'm not going to ask you to contemplate your navel and you can also forget any ideas of kaftan-clad figures chanting funny sounds and staring at candles. That is not what this book is about. Neither is it about tying yourself up in weird and agonising-looking positions. I am not going to ask you to stand on your head or to force your legs into the famous 'Lotus Position'. In fact you won't be forcing yourself to do anything!

What I have done is to take the very cleverly conceived ancient Yoga postures and adapt them into wonderfully-enjoyable slow, stretching movements that gently exercise the entire body. Nothing is pushed or forced and the feeling is one of languid indulgence. This is of course the opposite of what most of us have been taught – that in order to get and stay fit repetitive, exhausting exercise is the only route. In fact the phrase 'It has to hurt to do you good' is still heard today. While I think this could be applied to dancers or athletes who have to keep their bodies tuned to an exaggerated degree, for people leading normal lives who simply want to get and keep themselves fit, healthy, strong and supple, there is no need for that kind of punishing regime.

I am not dismissing completely 'physical jerks' as I believe they have their part to play. However, in my experience, the vast majority of people who embark on this type of energetic exercise programme, launch themselves into it with tremendous enthusiasm, only to give up weeks rather than months later. The simple truth is that exhausting repetitive exercises are not nice to do, and while you puff and pant and the sweat pours off you, you're praying that it will soon be over so you can crumple in a heap and convince yourself that it was all worth it. Add to this the usual accompaniment of pulled muscles, strained or torn ligaments and even misplaced joints on occasion, and the idea isn't too appealing. It is inevitable that the 'dreaded' workout is soon dropped.

In total contrast, these slow Yoga movements take no exertion, feel wonderful to do, cannot damage muscles, ligaments etc., and leave you feeling not only stretched, strong and supple, but also relaxed and revitalised as well. What's more, this style of Yoga can be perfectly integrated into your life to become your permanent regime.

I know it sounds too good to be true, but as you'll discover, it isn't.

ON THE PHYSICAL LEVEL

The key to the value of these movements is the fact that everything is done in slow motion. And when you move so slowly and smoothly you become acutely aware of your body and can stretch your ligaments and muscles to their limits, but in a totally controlled way. This control means that you are able to stop before there is any danger of pulling or straining anything which is of course quite the reverse of conventional exercise, where you move so quickly, that you only know you have done some damage afterwards, when unfortunately it is too late.

During each movement there is a point at which you stop, just for a few seconds, to hold your position still. This brief pause is sufficient to establish the necessary stretch, in what I call your 'natural limit position'. This 'natural limit position' is very important, and is obtained with absolutely no exertion or pushing whatsoever. You will know the instant you reach this point if you concentrate completely on what you are feeling and move slowly and smoothly as instructed, and this is where you stop. You then continue to the end of the movement, going into a specified relaxation position, so that your body can unwind completely before continuing with the next movement in the routine.

Competition is non-existent and therefore your 'natural limit position' does not have to be the same as anyone else's. Everyone's body **is** different and you are obtaining the absolute maximum benefit for yourself if you only go to your individual limit.

To illustrate this further, imagine standing, legs apart, relaxing your body over and forwards from the hips. When your arms and hands hang completely relaxed, without any pushing, your hands may be level with your knees. However, the person next to you could be comfortably relaxed over with his hands hanging level with his ankles. That does not mean that he is getting more benefit than you, just because it appears that he is going to a more advanced position. The benefit is derived from these Yoga movements when you don't try to go any further than your own natural limit because, having stopped and established the stretch in the holding position, the next time you repeat that movement your natural limit will have increased automatically and you will go further. Forget the theory that in life you must always try just that little bit harder, because with this way of moving and improving the body, it really doesn't apply.

It is also important to understand that you are not using *just* the muscles and joints involved during the actual holding period of these movements. Many additional areas of the body are being gently worked as you go into and out of the holding positions, and because the movements are slow and controlled,

these muscles and joints are strengthening and improving as well. Therefore, each movement gets to much more of the body than you might at first think and this is another reason why Yoga done this way is so valuable.

ON THE MENTAL LEVEL

People are always saying to me, 'I try so hard to relax and clear my mind but thoughts just keep swimming around in my head, and no matter what I do, I can't seem to stop them.' These Yoga movements will clear, relax and calm the mind as well as the body.

As you go slowly through each movement, your mind is totally concentrated and absorbed in what you are feeling and doing, and whether your mind likes it or not, all other thoughts and preoccupations are simply forced

out. This means that for the duration of the movement, you are completely indulging yourself in you and your sensations and feeling wonderful. At the end of the movement, you feel not only physically good and relaxed, but mentally at peace as well. When you know the movements by heart, you will find this mental absorption lasting right through your routine from beginning to end, but at first your attention may wander just a little between movements.

Many people find that after practising for a while, the tremendous mental relief and relaxation that they feel enables them to 'turn off' as they begin their routine, and sort of hang their lives on a hook together with all their worries, anxieties and frustrations. The effect of this is that afterwards there is often a

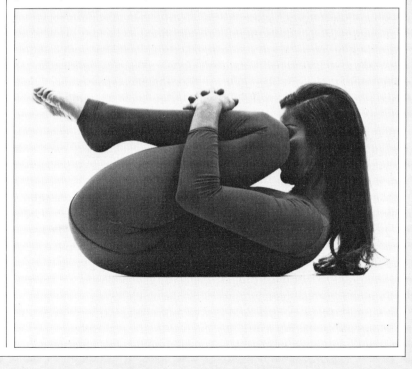

change of perspective, and instead of wasting valuable energy continuing to worry about problems and anxieties, this energy can be used constructively to actually do something about them.

When the mind is jumbled and confused, it is impossible to think clearly and decide what to do. This results, not surprisingly, in the problems going round and round in your head as you steadily become more and more neurotic. Once the mind has been completely cleared however it is much easier to be calmly selective and choose which of the problems or anxieties needs the most urgent attention, deal with it efficiently and go on to the next problem that needs sorting out.

Perhaps you are beginning to see just how important, and even vital to physical and mental health this ability to clear and relax the mind regularly is. It is not a luxury; it is a necessity.

HOW DOES THIS STYLE OF YOGA DIFFER FROM OTHER STYLES?

Hatha – which means physical – Yoga, is being widely practised today in the Western world and is becoming more and more popular as people discover its benefits.

With many styles of teaching Hatha Yoga, the finished posture or Asana, as it is called, is the most important part, and if you cannot attain the position at first, you work and strive towards it. With these *Everyday Yoga* movements on the other hand, there is no accent on a finished position or pose. The movements are continuous, with a very brief holding period half-way through in a pos-

ition that your body determines. There is no striving or working towards a specific position, and your body tells you when it is ready to go on rather than you telling it.

You may already have noticed that I refer to 'movements' rather than 'positions' or 'postures' and this is because each movement encompasses slowly going towards the holding position, a brief pause to establish the stretch, slowly coming out of the position and the subsequent relaxation position.

Another difference regarding styles of Yoga, is the speed with which the Asanas, or postures, are performed. Although compared to conventional exercise, most styles of Yoga are executed slowly, this style of Yoga is done even more slowly. If you think of 'slow', then think of 'extra slow', and then think of 'extra, extra slow', you will have more of an idea of the correct speed of the movements. It is this extremely slow, controlled way of moving that is different from many other styles of Yoga being taught today and which I feel is responsible for the additional side-benefits, emotional and mental as well as physical.

Indian Sanskrit is often used to teach the original names of the postures and techniques. My feeling, however, is that having to learn complicated-sounding ancient Indian words and phrases, is neither desirable nor necessary, and only causes confusion. Although it is true that the postures which evolved into these movements were established in the East, I see no practical reason why easily understandable and

remembered English names cannot be used. Therefore, as you will see, all the individual movements and breathing techniques in the book have English descriptive names.

WEIRD RITUALS

You may have been put off Yoga before by pictures of Yogis involved in extremely uncomfortable-looking cleansing rituals. One of these entails pushing great lengths of bandage up the nostrils and down into the intestines to clean them. Well, you can put the first-aid box away because, although I believe that these techniques were probably very necessary to cope with the health risks that abounded in Asia many years ago, most of us do not live on the banks of the River Ganges and therefore are not subject to the attendant dangers!

There is another technique designed to clear the sinuses, where salt water is sniffed up each nostril alternately. Sea water is favoured for this, so if you fancy a quick nip down to Southend that's fine, but once again, I don't feel that it's necessary to include this.

Also, there will be no walking on hot coals, or lying down for a quick nap on a bed of nails, and I am definitely not organising a package tour to the foothills of the Himalayas. To be serious though, maybe even today, in certain parts of the world, these seemingly curious and eccentric rituals are valuable, but here with our Western way of life, I feel we really do not need to include them.

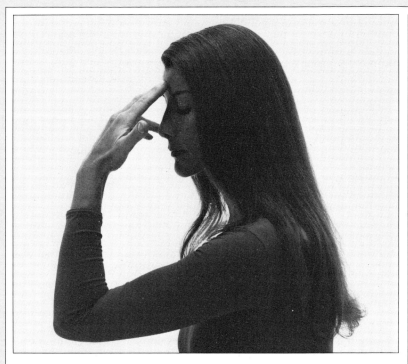

concentrated thought, with the effect of clearing all other superfluous thoughts from the mind. This is exactly what is happening in your mind as you go through the Yoga movements. You are involved in a form of meditation and receiving the benefits of that meditation – namely a clear and relaxed mind – every time you go through your practice routine.

PHILOSOPHY – NECESSARY OR NOT?

Many people are afraid that getting involved with Yoga means that they will have to study and adopt the philosophy of Yoga as well. Nothing could be further from the truth. Although I feel that parts of the Yogic philosophy are not only relevant to our lives today but also extremely valuable and fascinating, I do not see it as either a prerequisite or necessary accompaniment to the wonderfully beneficial practice of the movements.

My main concern is that as many people as possible simply **use** this way of moving the body to improve their lives right now – today! The reasons for starting are unimportant – I am as happy to see the man suffering from back ache or worried about his falling hair, as the man who wants to begin Yoga to raise his spiritual consciousness.

There are many people who, after being introduced to Hatha or physical Yoga, do wish to get involved with the philosophy, but in my experience, very many more don't. They simply enjoy what they get out of their practice and the benefit they feel in their lives as a result, and don't

YOGA BREATHING

Breathing is a very important part of Yoga practice, and many people mistakenly assume that they are going to have to learn complex breathing techniques. Don't worry – the kind of breathing we are going to do is quite straightforward, totally uncomplicated and very easy to learn.

It is simply a question of breathing in and out at the correct times during the movement, so that your breathing works for you and not against you. You also get used to taking slightly deeper breaths than usual, and this not only helps the execution of the movements, but improves your breathing and lung capacity in your everyday life.

As you will see, the complete breathing instruction is added only when you know the movement, so that you can concentrate on what your body is doing first.

There are one or two other breathing techniques contained in the routine, but these are also extremely simple, and you will have no trouble following the instructions when you come to them.

MEDITATION

The word meditation often conjures up images of people sitting cross-legged, chanting 'Mantras' or special sounds that bring them to a state of meditation. Other people use the flame of a candle, stare at a design, or think of a particular image to do the same thing. While you will not be doing that kind of separate meditation, you are actually in a state of meditation as you go through the routine.

You see meditation means

want to take it any further.

The choice, therefore, is yours.

TENSION AND ANXIETY – SPECIFIC REMEDIES

Acute tension and anxiety cause many of today's problems. Hypertension, insomnia, coronary heart disease, migraine, intestinal disorders and asthma are just a few of the more well-known conditions, and there are many more. Learning how you can diffuse and eliminate tension when it occurs in your life is therefore very valuable.

As well as the general clearing and relaxation of the mind brought about by regular practice of the routine, there are specific movements and techniques contained in the book that can be used individually in everyday life situations when you are feeling particularly tense or nervous,

and you will find these extremely useful.

Among these special remedy techniques, there is one that I call a 'Natural Tranquilliser'. Its real name is the Alternate Nostril Breathing technique, and you will find it on page 44. This is a very potent relaxant, and has been used with great success to help sufferers from insomnia and migraine. It can also be used whenever you find yourself becoming nervous or edgy and need to calm yourself down instantly, or simply to clear your head and improve your breathing.

Another wonderful movement in terms of the results it brings, is shown here. It's called the Tension Release, page 82. This is especially good for people who develop that sometimes excruciating pain right at the top of the back. This is often the case

with people who spend a large part of their day bending over to work, and if you are prone to this type of tension pain, simply execute the Tension Release movement slowly once or twice. The relief is quite dramatic. Wherever you happen to be, just find a quiet corner and take three or four minutes to do it.

A third important relaxation-inducer in the book, that amongst other things, eliminates the stiffness and tension in the neck that so many people suffer, is called the Head Roll, and you will find it on page 48. Follow the instructions carefully, and even though you may be doing it in the middle of a busy working day, do it smoothly and slowly. It takes only three or four minutes of your time and you will relieve the stiffness, pain and tension.

With all of the above movements, you have no need to change your clothing, but make sure that there is nothing too tight or restricting around the waist or neck.

IS THERE AN AGE LIMIT?

No, my students range in age from eight to eighty. The extreme gentleness of this style of Yoga makes it the ideal form of body movement for people of all ages.

Many people who are unfit because of lack of exercise over many years find this style of Yoga not only easy and enjoyable to do, but immediately effective in improving their health and strength.

At the other end of the scale, you may find that your children want to practise the routine with you. This is fine as long as they are mature enough to be able to

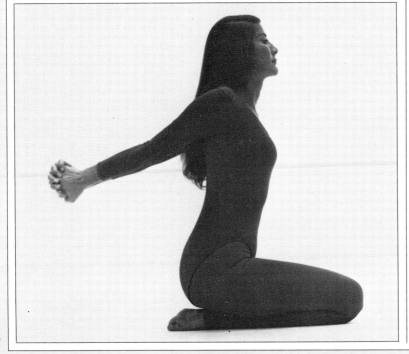

concentrate on what they are doing without distracting you.

WILL I HAVE TO BECOME A VEGETARIAN?

Although people are becoming increasingly aware of the benefits and advantages of being vegetarian and feel happier and healthier because of it there is absolutely no reason why you should become one unless you wish to do so. I should add, however, that positive changes often occur in your eating and drinking habits through the practice of Yoga for the following reasons.

Because the Yoga movements are performed slowly and smoothly, never rushing with anything, the same feeling often washes over into other areas of your life that you didn't necessarily think about before. Eating is one of those areas, and many people who used to wolf their food down, hardly tasting it, find that they take more time to relax when eating, and savour each mouthful before swallowing it. Doctors will tell you that the digestive process starts in the mouth with mastication and therefore the longer the food stays there the better.

Your taste buds also become more alive, especially with regular practice of movements such as the Lion and the Jaw Lift (see page 40) and many people go off certain foods and develop preferences for others. What I find remarkable is the consistent uniformity in the dietary changes of my students over the years.

One of the first things that people usually go off is red meat, preferring the taste of white meat or fish. As many doctors and nutritionists feel that red meat is too rich in fat for a healthy diet, this change is all to the good. Another common occurrence is that people go off heavily-spiced and seasoned food and thick sauces, wanting to taste the actual food itself rather than the condiments, and many start eating simple unadorned meals, appreciating the taste of certain foods for the first time. The consumption of coffee and alcohol often diminishes too, and, like the other changes, though not intentionally brought about, are certainly healthy.

Perhaps, when you are ready, some of these changes will happen to you, but don't force it. Cutting out certain foods because you have lost the taste for them is very different from depriving yourself of foods that you like. The latter will only cause resentment, so wait until it happens naturally.

HOW ABOUT SMOKING?

To smoke or not to smoke has been a controversial issue for some time now, but I feel that the accumulated medical evidence certainly shows that smoking cannot be considered healthy.

Smoking is not an easy habit to break, especially if you are addicted to nicotine and have smoked for many years, but many people have successfully given up smoking through the practice of Yoga.

Like many other habits, smoking is a prop – a comforter in times of insecurity – and it is not just the smoking itself which is important but the entire ritual surrounding it. There is a feeling of safety in the familiarity of this ritual and many smokers are nervous about eliminating it. What, they feel, would take its place?

With regular practice of Yoga several things happen. Nerves are calmed, anxiety and tension are eliminated, and you become a much more physically and mentally-relaxed person generally. There is a moment of decision when you actually choose to smoke that cigarette or not, and the more agitated and tense you are, the more likely you are to light it. If, on the other hand, you are already calm, and can rationally decide, 'Do I really need this cigarette?' before lighting up, the decision will often go the other way, and this, smokers say, can be the turning point.

Another way of using Yoga, is to go through one of the specific relaxation and tension-removing techniques or one of the breathing exercises, whenever you desperately want a cigarette. Not only will you feel calmer afterwards, but your self esteem will be greatly inflated because you used yourself and not an outside prop to get you through the moment.

Previously heavy smokers also say that the improved breathing which comes with regular practice of the movements makes the lungs feel so good and healthy that they don't want to counteract this by polluting them with nicotine. Many ex-smokers also notice a dramatic increase in physical ability in their lives generally, where they used to suffer shortness of breath.

If you are a smoker and sincerely want to give it up, try the relaxation and breathing techniques on pages 22, 24, 44, 48 and 82 – they really can help.

WILL I LOSE WEIGHT WITH YOGA?

If you have excess weight, you will definitely lose it with regular practice of the routine. More important than the actual weight loss however is the fact that there will be a noticeable reduction in inches as your muscles firm and tighten.

An additional aid to weight loss is the fact that certain movements stimulate the thyroid gland and it is the thyroid that is responsible for the efficiency of the metabolism.

Improved digestion and elimination of food are two other factors that contribute greatly to weight loss and adjustment.

CAN I SPOT-REDUCE WITH YOGA?

It seems to be an unfortunate fact of life that we put on weight in specific areas of the body. Generally speaking, these 'problem' areas seem loath to budge with diet and normal exercise. These areas are bottom, hips, tummy and thighs for women and the gut for men.

The regular practice of the Yoga routine will reduce these areas anyway, but if you feel your problem is more urgent don't despair, help is at hand. Certain of the movements in this book can be performed just on their own several times a day, to spot-reduce these 'problem' areas, and you will find which movements to do for which parts of your body in the glossary on page 89. Perform these movements two

or three times a day for quick results, but moving slowly and smoothly and following the instructions carefully.

CAN I DEVELOP CERTAIN AREAS OF MY BODY?

Yes, as with the above, there are specific movements which, if practised frequently, will develop certain areas of the body. This is useful if you feel that you have a particular weakness in, say, the shoulders, or the legs, or you want to develop the chest area.

Check in the glossary on page 89 for which movements to do and then try to perform them two or three times a day following the instructions.

WHAT ABOUT BACK PROBLEMS?

Back problems affect an enormous section of the population and it seems that little is known by the medical profession about how to cure them. Osteopaths are sometimes able to manipulate the joints in the back to bring some relief but for many people pain-killing tablets and rest are the only unsatisfactory solutions. More work days are apparently lost through 'back problems' than any other common condition, and the crippling effect of a bad back is both ageing and debilitating, so it is worth thinking not only about the cure but also the prevention.

Unless you have a bad back caused by a specific injury, you must take the responsibility for getting and keeping your back strong and healthy. This is not difficult. You simply need to gently flex your spine backwards

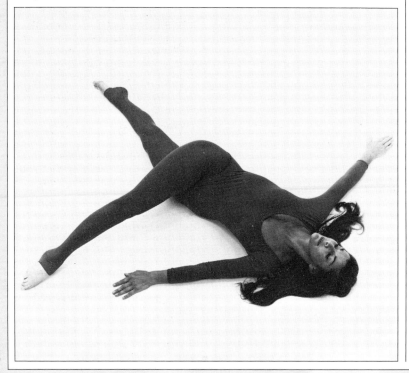

and forwards regularly in order to introduce, and then maintain, the suppleness and strength needed, so that your back is prepared for the sudden movements and strain that it is subjected to in everyday life, and that all too often lead to those misplaced joints and pulled muscles in an unhealthy back.

Just simply going through the routine in this book every day will ensure that your back is getting the correct movement, but if you cannot manage this, then pick out one or two of the specific back movements recommended in the glossary on page 89 and do these every day or as often as you can. The golden rule is to move your back both ways, slowly and gently, arching it and then hollowing it. If you do this, you should never have any back trouble.

Another golden rule for avoiding back problems, is never to curve your back when bending down to pick up something from the floor. Always go down with a straight back. This is easier to do with the legs apart, bending the knees outwards, and is therefore more comfortable for men or women wearing trousers. However it is possible for women in skirts to bend down with the knees together still keeping the back straight, even though it may feel a little strange at first. Think about your back each time you bend down for something and in a little while you will get used to doing it with your back straight. The effort is well worth it for a life free from back pains and problems.

Another valuable tip is to be aware of how you are sitting. Most of the chairs we sit on are

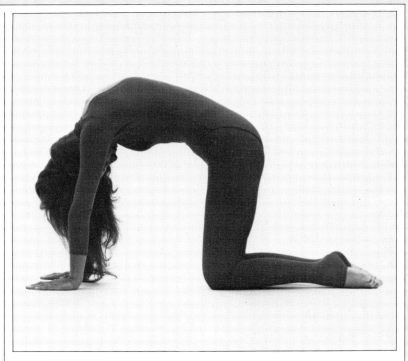

not designed with the health of the back in mind, especially the lounge chairs most of us have at home. We tend to slouch in these with the back curved and all the weight on the base of the spine putting a lot of strain on it. Try to sit as straight as you can, using cushions if necessary to help or, better still, don't spend long periods relaxing on these lounge chairs without getting up and stretching. Watching television is a particular instance when this can happen.

Lastly, a word about beds and sleeping positions: the more back support you get in bed the better, so a firm mattress rather than a soft one should be the rule, and one that gives your body even support. On the question of pillows I would recommend that only one and not too bulky a pillow be used. Any more than

that and the top of your spine is bent at an exaggerated angle causing unnecessary strain.*

The best position to sleep in is the position of Deep Relaxation shown on page 23 (used to relax at the beginning and end of your routine). Literally every muscle and joint is relaxed in this position and your breathing apparatus is completely free for the deep, even breathing that you need for sound and refreshing sleep.

Many people tell me that they have always slept curled up on

*__Note:__ This does not apply to people suffering from conditions such as hiatus hernia where it is not advisable to sleep with the body too flat, and sometimes two or more pillows are recommended.

their sides, and that they will never be able to sleep in this relaxation position. With regular practice of the routine, however, it often happens that the relaxation position becomes more and more comfortable, and it is then possible to adopt it for sleeping. To help you towards this, you might like to try using the mental relaxation technique while lying in the Deep Relaxation position in bed (see page 23) as this often gets you accustomed to the position very quickly.

COMMON CONDITIONS AND AILMENTS HELPED

With regular practice, Yoga can bring great relief and sometimes even complete elimination of many of today's common conditions and ailments, and although several of these have already been mentioned in the book, I have included them again here so that you have a very comprehensive check list.

For the following conditions use the movements and techniques on the page numbers indicated.

Acne and other skin disorders
Pages 28, 32, 38, 74

Hair loss and balding
Page 46

Migraine
Page 44

Indigestion
Page 84

Flatulence
Page 34

Constipation
Page 81

Overweight
Pages 30, 60, 64, 69

Insomnia
Pages 22, 44

Pre-menstrual tension
Page 84

Dysmenorrhoea
Page 84

Respiratory problems
Pages 24, 30, 44

Hypertension
Page 22

Sinusitis
Page 44

Eye strain
Page 50

Fatigue
Pages 24, 28, 44, 48, 64, 74

Bronchial conditions
Pages 22, 24

Varicose veins
Page 64

Headache
Pages 44, 48

Backache
Pages 28, 32, 34, 69, 74, 76, 84

Tension at top of back
Pages 28, 32, 76, 82

Tension in neck
Pages 28, 32, 34, 48, 76, 82

Asthmatic conditions
Page 44

Nasal catarrh
Page 44

Stiffening of the joints
Pages 38, 52, 53, 54, 56

Bad circulation
Pages 28, 38, 64, 74

Nervous conditions such as:

Nail biting
Page 44

Stuttering
Page 44

Nausea
Page 44

Agoraphobia
Page 44

Claustrophobia
Page 44

MEDICAL CAUTION

Although it is clear that Yoga improves your health and can be extremely therapeutic when used for many conditions, **it must never be used as a substitute for medical treatment.** If you are suffering from an illness or have a history of serious illness, you must check with your own doctor before commencing the routine. He knows your personal medical history and therefore is qualified to tell you whether you can safely undertake these movements.

More and more doctors are suggesting Yoga to their patients, especially in cases where people must not or cannot undertake strenuous exercise. I not only count many doctors amongst my students but have a steady flow of students referred to me by their doctors.

If your doctor isn't familiar with this slow gentle style of Yoga, show him the book so that he can see the kind of movements that you would be practising, and I am sure you will find him sympathetic.

PRACTICE

HOW TO PRACTISE WITH YOUR EVERYDAY ROUTINE

As you will see, there are fifteen main practice sections, beginning on page 22 – clearly numbered 1–15, and it is these fifteen sections that comprise your regular routine. There are also a further five sections that are lettered A–E. Do not worry about this second group for now; they are alternative movements that can be used after the main routine has been practised for quite a while, interchanging them with specific movements from the original routine. This is explained more fully on page 72.

Each practice session starts and ends with a specified period in the position of Deep Relaxation, as shown at the beginning of Section 1. This relaxation period is very important as it enables you to begin your routine with a more relaxed body and mind. Take particular note of it and try not to cut it short. The same relaxation position is also adopted at the end of your routine.

After the period of Deep Relaxation, you are ready to begin. However, don't simply look at the pictures and assume that you know how to do the movements. Essential details such as the precise positioning of fingers, hands, elbows, feet etc., and the exact order of every facet of the movement are vitally important.

It is rare for these movements to exercise only one area of the body; more usually several parts are involved. If you wish to reap the potential rewards of each movement to the full, take a little time to read and absorb the information and instructions given before you actually start to practise.

Begin with Section 1, on page 22, and practise **only** this section until you feel absolutely comfortable with it and know the movements by heart without referring to the pictures or captions. Then practise Sections 1 and 2 together. Continue practising 1 and 2 until once again you feel absolutely sure of what you are doing and know the movements by heart, and then practise Sections 1, 2 and 3 together. In this way gradually work through until you are practising all fifteen Sections, and the complete routine.

It doesn't matter how long you spend practising each additional section of the routine. It could be days, weeks or even months. You will be receiving the benefit from the moment you begin your first session, so don't rush to do the completed routine, and be honest with yourself about really knowing what you are doing before going on.

HOW OFTEN SHOULD I PRACTISE?

This book may be called *Everyday Yoga* but that does not mean that you must go through the entire routine every single day. Everybody's life is different, and how often you practise will depend on how you fit your practice into your lifestyle. There are several ways of doing this, as you will see from the following questions and answers. Decide after reading them which suits you best.

HOW LONG DOES THE ROUTINE TAKE?

If the entire routine is done at the correct speed, working slowly and smoothly, the actual movements themselves should take approximately 45–60 minutes. Add on to this 5–8 minutes of deep relaxation both at the beginning and at the end of your routine, and you get a total of approximately an hour to an hour and a quarter for the whole session.

CAN I DO THE ROUTINE EVERY DAY?

If you are one of the lucky people

who have the time to do the routine every day, that is wonderful. Try not to cut down on the recommended times if you can, even though it may seem strange to move so slowly at first. As you get to know the movements more and start to really enjoy them, you may find that you are actually wanting to take longer over them. Well, the slower you do them, the more you will be getting out of them, so if you have the time, indulge.

WHAT ARE THE ALTERNATIVES TO EVERYDAY PRACTICE OF THE ROUTINE?

If you can't do the Routine every day, and many people find this impossible, pick out two or three days a week on which to practise and try to stick to the same days each week if you can. Alternatively, if you are really very short of time, do the routine once a week, but make sure that you do it on a day when you can really give time to yourself, with absolutely no rushing.

Obviously, the more often you practise and the more regularly, the better, but that doesn't mean doing the routine every day, and rushing through it, is going to benefit you as much as doing it at your leisure once, twice or three times a week.

CAN I DO SHORTER VERSIONS OF THE ROUTINE?

Yes, if you cannot manage to take the time for the whole routine, then it is possible to do a contracted version. In order to do this, some of the movements in the routine have to be eliminated with care, so that the remaining movements still give the overall head-to-toe benefit of the fuller routine.

I have worked out some shorter routines for you taking 20, 30 and 40 minutes, and these are on pages 86, 87 and 88.

You may like the idea of doing a short routine twice a day instead of the longer one only once a day, or using shorter routines two or three times a week, saving the complete routine for when you are not so rushed.

Use both the short and long routines in a way that suits your way of life best.

Note: You may reduce the time spent in the position of Deep Relaxation to four minutes when doing the shorter routines.

WHAT TIME OF DAY SHOULD I PRACTISE?

The time of day isn't actually that important. What will determine the time of day however, is the fact that you should never practise after a big meal, and in fact it is better not to have eaten for two and a half to three hours. The reasons for this are very logical. After eating, your body's energy is directed towards the digestion of the food and this happens quite naturally. If you force your body to divert some of this energy to the bending and stretching of your Yoga practice, you are creating an internal war and only succeeding in depleting the body's energy for both of the tasks that it has to perform. Subsequently, both will suffer. Remember, Yoga is about listen-

ing to the body and using the energy in as natural and positive a way as possible. On a simpler note, if your stomach is full, it just doesn't feel good to bend and stretch the body around.

Regarding light snacks and drinks, you do not need to wait for two and a half to three hours before you practise, but I do recommend at least thirty to sixty minutes.

The rule about eating, is always to eat after your routine wherever possible, and if you must eat before, make it as light as you can. The eating rule means that the obvious best times to practise are in the morning before breakfast, or prior to your evening meal, or late at night before going to bed. Try practising at different times of the day and see what time suits you best.

WHERE SHOULD I PRACTISE?

Try to practise somewhere quiet where you won't be disturbed, so that you can completely concentrate on what you are doing.

This is your Yoga period, and I want you to indulge yourself in you – at least for the duration of your session. Unless you live alone, it may mean that uninterrupted time to yourself is a luxury not easily obtained. However, if you make it absolutely clear to the people or family around you how important it is that you are not to be disturbed, hopefully you will be listened to. As a last resort, lock yourself away in the bedroom.

Whichever room you practise in, make sure that there is enough space to lie down on the floor in comfort, so that when you stretch your arms out at your sides you do not hit the furniture.

Try, if possible, to have some fresh air coming into the room. You are going to be taking deep breaths and increasing your intake of air and oxygen, so make it as fresh as possible.

CAN I PRACTISE IN THE OPEN AIR, WEATHER PERMITTING?

Practising your Yoga routine in the open air can be the most beneficial way to do it. However, there are some important points to remember regarding this.

The temperature has to be sufficiently hot so that you are comfortable not only doing the movements but also when you are lying down for the relaxation periods at the beginning and end of your session. The body cools down very quickly when it is horizontal, and if you are cold, it will prevent you from relaxing properly and subsequently devalue the entire routine.

Conversely, if you are in a hot climate, practise either early or late in the day, but never in the heat of the midday sun. High temperatures deplete the energy and you will not get the best from your practice.

It is very easy to be distracted in a garden or on a beach etc., where there are things going on around you. You need to be totally aware of only yourself and usually you have more chance of this in a controlled environment like your home. So consider these points carefully.

Another important point about practising in the open air is the surface. You need to have a flat, straight surface on which to do your Yoga, so that you have the correct balance and control. If the ground is uneven, you could hurt yourself. The best way to practise out of doors is on a terrace or patio, where you have access to fresh air but where the floor surface is perfectly flat.

DO I NEED A SPECIAL YOGA MAT?

An ideal floor surface for practice is a carpet or rug that does not move about, and if you have these at home, then that is fine.

The most important thing when practising the standing movements is that your feet grip, giving you a very stable position, and you can test this by standing with the legs apart, as for the Triangle on page 30. If your feet slip apart even slightly you need another non-slip surface on your existing carpet or rug. A towel can be used for this purpose or better still, a rubber-backed Yoga mat.

You may like to practise with bare feet, and this is fine. However, never practise on a stone or marble floor without using a Yoga mat or some other substantial floor covering as this can be potentially harmful to your kidneys.

WHAT SHOULD I WEAR TO PRACTISE?

Clothes generally inhibit body movement, and if you are alone and have assured privacy, then wear nothing or as little clothing as possible. If you feel more comfortable with something on, then wear clothes that give you complete freedom of movement in every direction, and make absolutely sure that there is nothing tight or restricting around the waist to limit your breathing. For this reason elasticated waistbands are best on shorts or track suit trousers, and most men find either of these good to work in. Women can wear shorts, track suits or leotards, whichever feels the most comfortable.

CAN I DO THE ROUTINE WITH A GROUP OF FRIENDS?

Yes, but make sure that everyone in the group has enough room for both the standing and lying movements without needing to constantly change position, as this will be distracting.

Once you start the routine, do it together, but try not to chat amongst yourselves. You need to concentrate completely on what you personally are doing and feeling to get the maximum benefit.

CAN I DO ANY HARM TO MYSELF?

In my thirteen years of teaching, I can honestly say that not one of my students has ever suffered a pulled muscle or ligament or indeed done any damage of any description.

With this slow, controlled style of Yoga, if you are heeding the instructions and doing the movements correctly, it is virtually impossible to hurt yourself.

A word of caution however. If you are currently suffering from any injury or illness, you must check with your doctor before you begin to practise.

PRACTICE SECTIONS 1-15

THE ROUTINE

SECTION 1

POSITION OF DEEP RELAXATION

The position of Deep Relaxation is exactly what it says it is, a position in which you are able literally to relax all of your muscles and, very importantly, your mind as well.

As you will see, it is not simply a question of lying down on the floor and closing your eyes. The positioning of the head, hands and feet, is very important if you are to get maximum relaxation.

The correct position, combined with the mind-clearing technique described below, prepares you perfectly for your routine, and enables you to concentrate easily and completely on each movement as you come to it. The relaxation period after your routine allows you to really indulge and let your body go after the gentle stretches that you have been putting it through, and it also gives you the time to prepare yourself mentally to return to your day's activities.

Ideally, you should relax in this position for between five and eight minutes both before and after your routine. However, if you absolutely must cut down the time try to go no lower than four minutes for each relaxation period otherwise you will affect the potential of the routine.

Note: This limit of four minutes also applies with the shortened routines, see page 86.

As well as using the position of Deep Relaxation at the beginning and end of your routine, it can be used entirely on its own, whenever you feel in need of complete relaxation. This applies particularly to people who have difficulty in sleeping and the position used with the mind-clearing technique, has been known to put a speedy end to restless nights.

MIND CLEARING TECHNIQUE

1 Lie down slowly until you are flat on your back. Allow your legs and feet to gently fall open. Rest your hands on the floor palms uppermost, and let your fingers curl. Close your eyes, and gently tilt your head back until you feel a slight suggestion of a stretch at the front of your throat.

Now you are ready to begin the mind-clearing technique.

Don't move a muscle, just imagine that you are looking at a photograph of yourself lying in the position of deep relaxation.

Gradually work up the body mentally, following the numbers, imagining in detail how each part of you looks. Keep each image in your mind for approximately twenty seconds before moving on.

After you have learned the order in which to work through the body, keep your eyes closed so that you can concentrate completely on the images in your mind.

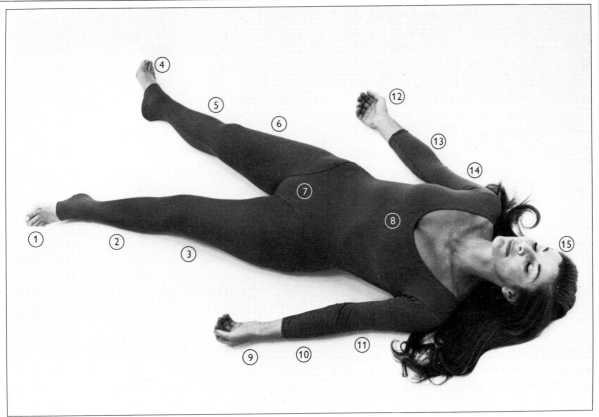

1	Begin with the left foot.	**6**	Right thigh.	**11**	Left upperarm.
2	Left calf.	**7**	Abdominal area.	**12**	Right hand.
3	Left thigh.	**8**	Chest area.	**13**	Right forearm.
4	Right foot.	**9**	Left hand.	**14**	Right upperarm.
5	Right calf.	**10**	Left forearm.	**15**	All of the face.

AN ADDITIONAL WORD ABOUT BREATHING

With the majority of movements in the routine, you will see that I instruct you simply to take a deep breath at the beginning of the movement. Take that initial breath, when indicated, and then just forget about the breath and let your body breathe naturally, concentrating your mind on what you are doing.

After you have practised the routine for a while and know the movements by heart you can, if you wish, incorporate the more complex breathing instructions given in the tinted boxes with each movement.

There are a few movements contained in the routine where specific breathing instructions must be followed from the very beginning, and in these cases, I have included the correct breathing procedure in the general instructions.

Note: As a rule, all the breathing in your routine is done through the nose.

COMPLETE BREATH

During the Deep Relaxation period, your breathing has become slower and more relaxed, so we begin the routine with some deep breaths to wake the lungs up and to get used to taking larger and deeper breaths. The Complete Breath movement also starts to gently stretch the back, arms and sides of the body.

The movement entails simply raising and lowering the arms at your sides, inhaling to a count of four as you raise, and exhaling to a count of four as you lower.

Count to yourself at approximately the same speed as seconds.

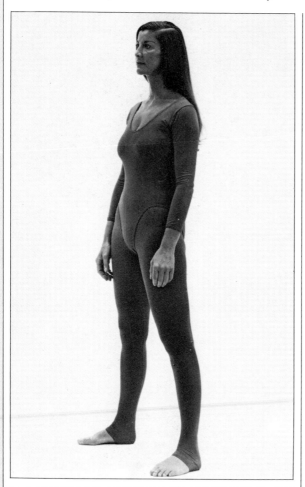

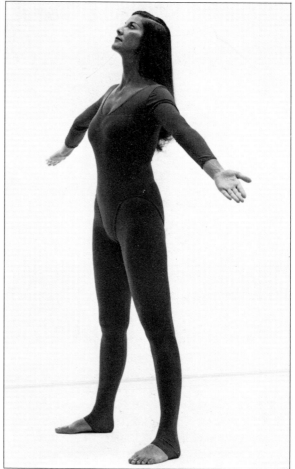

1 Stand with your legs and feet about two feet apart, making sure that your toes point straight in front of you and not out to the side.
  Let your arms and hands relax at your sides.

2 Inhale deeply through the nose to the count of four and raise the arms at the same time. Keep the elbows straight and palms uppermost as you raise.

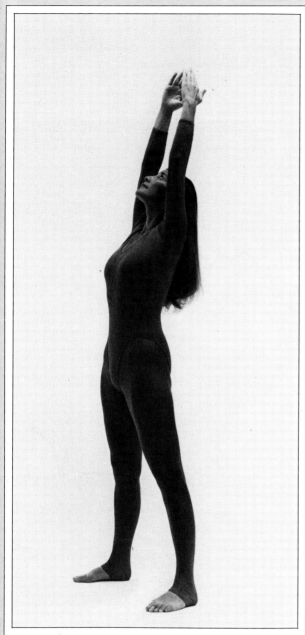

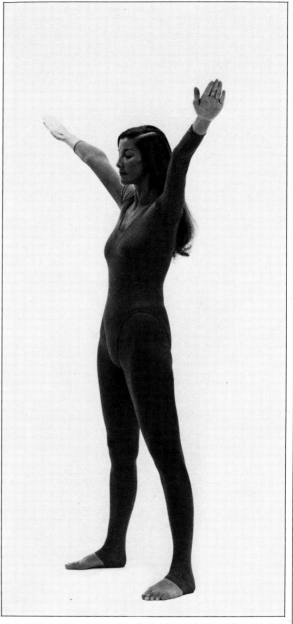

3 Try to bring your fingertips together, looking up to see the ceiling. Really stretch up.

4 Exhale slowly, to the count of four lowering the arms at the same time. Relax for just a moment, then repeat raising and lowering movement a further three times.

   Stay in your position ready to go on to the next movement.

STANDING STRETCH INTO THE REFRESHER

The Standing Stretch is a continuous movement that gently warms the body up in preparation for the routine.

The body is stretched forward, backward and side to side, and then relaxed over in the Refresher position (see page 28).

To begin with, bend the body only to the most moderate positions shown.

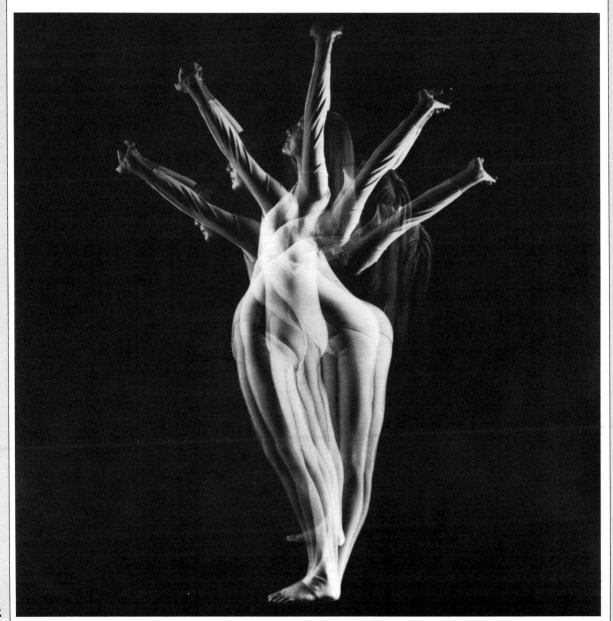

1 *Left* Interlock the fingers and push the hands up. Bend slowly forward and then back from the hips.

2 Let your hips sway over to your left and bend the top of your body to the right, but only to a moderate angle at first. Straighten up smoothly and repeat to the left side.

Breathing:
Inhale when upright in starting position.
Exhale as you bend forwards.
Inhale as you straighten up again.
Exhale when upright ready to repeat for back bend and side to side bends.

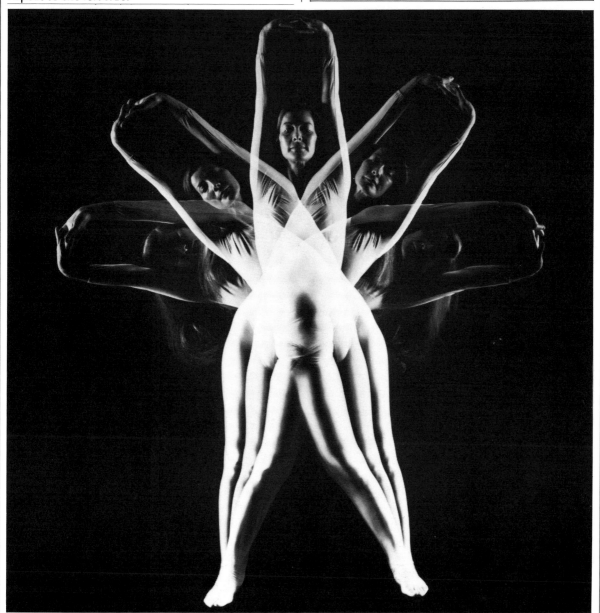

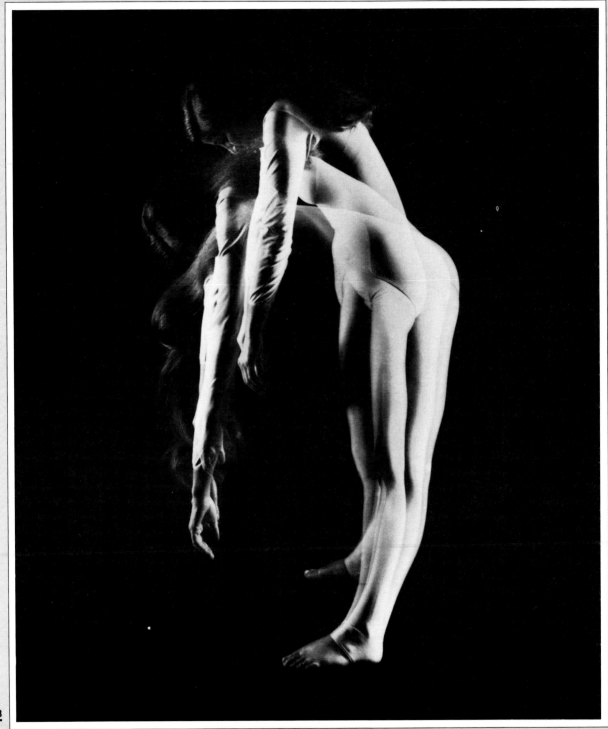

THE REFRESHER

This is the relaxation position used at the end of the Standing Stretch, as well as some other standing movements in the routine. However, it is so valuable in its own right that to regard it as just a resting position at the end of a movement is to do it a grave injustice.

The Refresher not only refreshes by increasing the blood flow into the head and face, but it also relaxes the neck, shoulders, arms and hands. Its true potential, however, is the way in which it quickly establishes an extraordinary amount of strength and suppleness in the back and spine. This occurs during the slow uncoiling of the body as it straightens up, as each vertebra in turn is forced to take part in the controlled, smooth raising of the body. This has the effect of not only strengthening the spine but also the muscles on either side of the spine.

When you do the Refresher, close your eyes and concentrate on uncoiling your back as slowly and as smoothly as you can, not raising your head until your back is straight, and then waiting a few seconds before opening your eyes.

Relax over gently from the hips, allowing the weight of your head, arms and hands to bring you to your 'natural' limit without any pushing. Then slowly uncoil the back, bringing your head up last of all.

SECTION 2

THE TRIANGLE INTO THE REFRESHER

The Triangle really gives the sides of the body a good but gentle stretch, slimming and firming the sides and the waist. It also strengthens the arms, shoulders, leg muscles and back, and expands the chest and improves balance and co-ordination.

When you bend over to take your leg, make sure that you grip it just below the knee rather than on the knee. You need a good grip so that you can lean your body weight on to the leg for the holding period, in order to establish the correct stretch in your side, see picture 4.

Don't let your shoulders, hips or head twist as you go to the side; keep them all square to the front.

Breathing:
Inhale as arms are raised.
Exhale bending over to side.
Inhale straightening up again.
Exhale as arms are lowered to sides.

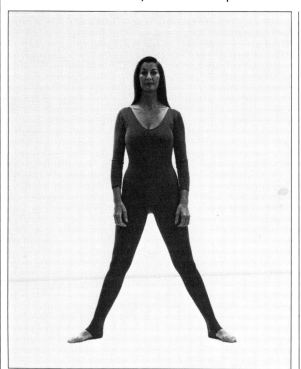

1 Stand with the legs and feet 2–2½ ft. apart, turning the toes out to the side. Relax the shoulders, arms and hands.

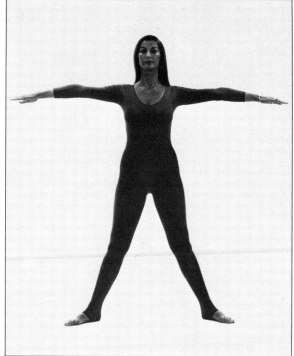

2 Inhale deeply as you raise the arms to shoulder level.

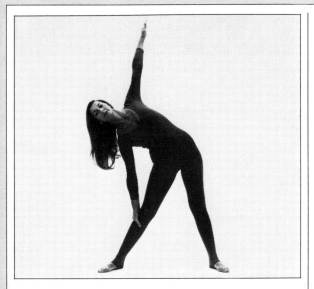

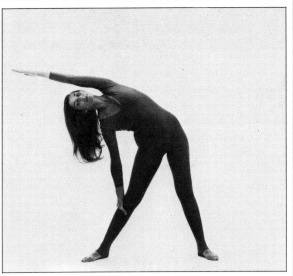

3 Bend slowly and smoothly to your right, and grip the right leg just below the knee.

4 Bring the left arm over towards the ear, keeping the elbow as straight as you can and turning the palm towards the floor. Hold the position still for a count of five, counting to yourself at approximately the same speed as seconds.

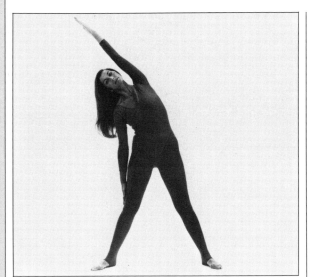

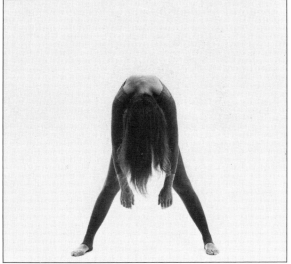

5 Straighten up to position 2, then lower the arms and relax the head, shoulders, arms and hands as in position 1. Repeat to left side, and then once again on both sides.

6 Relax forward from the hips in the Refresher position, uncoiling the back slowly as with the previous movement.

THE FISH

Many of the Yoga movements work on increasing the strength and suppleness of the spine, and the Fish does this by gently arching the back upwards.

As well as working on the back the Fish strengthens the neck, arms and shoulders. It also increases the blood flow into the head and face, refreshing them.

Try not to jerk as you arch the back, and aim for a raise of just a few inches at first. Hold your arched position still for the count of five, and then indulge yourself in the last part of the movement by letting your head slide back as slowly as you can.

As soon as you know the movement, do it with your eyes closed. You will find it a powerful relaxation-inducer.

Note: If your head does not slide back easily, see picture 4, place a silky scarf under your head before you begin.

Breathing:
Inhale as for position 3.
Exhale during the count.
Inhale as the back sinks down.
Exhale when the back is flat on the floor again.

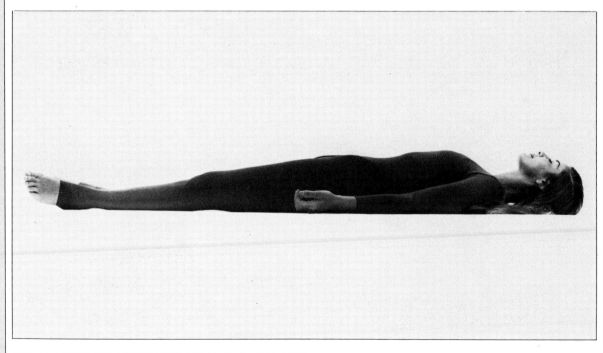

1 Lie down slowly, flat on your back and relax in the position of Deep Relaxation.

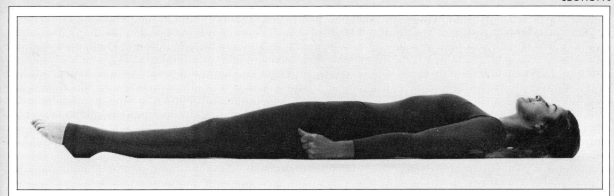

2 Close the legs and feet and make fists of the hands with the thumbs uppermost.

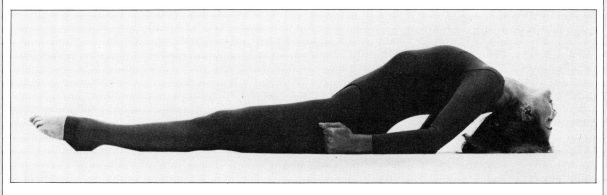

3 Inhale deeply through the nose, push down with the elbows and fists, and gently arch the back by pushing the chest up and letting the head tilt back. Hold your position for a count of five.

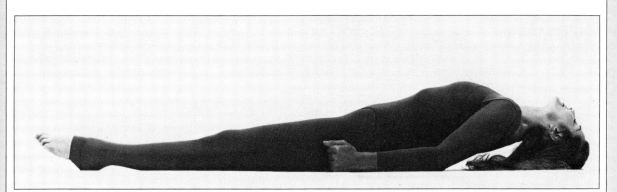

4 Allow your head to slide slowly back, without pushing it, and when your back is flat on the floor again, let your legs and feet fall open, rest your hands on their backs, let your fingers curl, keep your eyes closed, and rest for a few moments. Then repeat once more. Do the movement twice at first and increase gradually to four times.

SECTION 4

THE COIL

The Coil is the counterpart of the preceding Fish movement in that it bends the back in completely the opposite direction, giving it a lovely stretch from the base, right to the top of the spine.

The Coil not only works the spine, but also strengthens and eliminates stiffness from the neck and increases strength in the arms and shoulders. It also firms up the buttocks.

Do not try to touch your knees with your forehead when you start. The objective is to bend the knees in and then bring your head towards the knees, so that you come into a position that you can hold still comfortably for the count of five. In time, your head will come closer and closer to your knees until eventually they may touch, but that is not the initial aim.

Try not to jerk with any part of the movement; keep it slow and controlled.

Breathing:
Inhale as for position 2.
Exhale as head is brought towards knees.
Inhale as head goes back to floor.
Exhale as head touches floor.

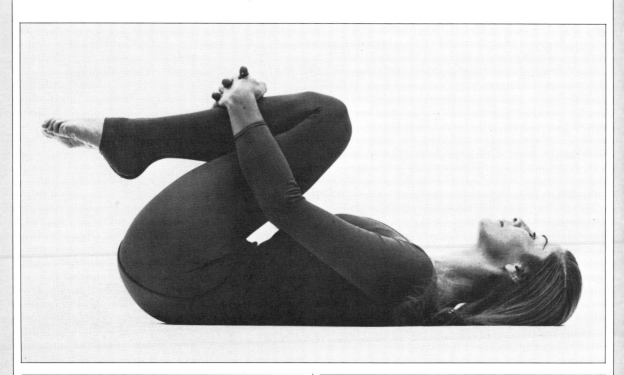

1 Relax for a few moments in the position of Deep Relaxation, then bring the legs and feet together and bend the knees in towards your chest. Inter-lock your fingers and loop the hands over the knees, about mid-calf.

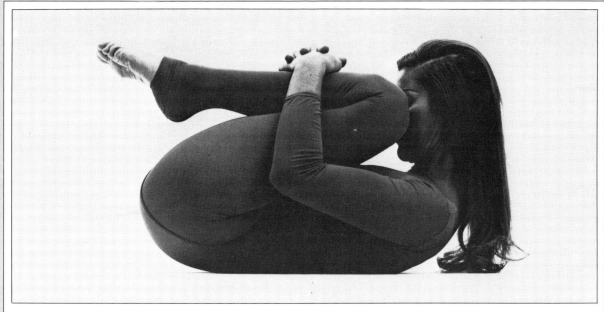

2 Inhale deeply, and smoothly pull the knees closer into your chest. Then raise your head with control and bring it slowly towards your knees, stopping in a comfortable position. In time your forehead may touch your knees as shown.
Hold for a count of five.

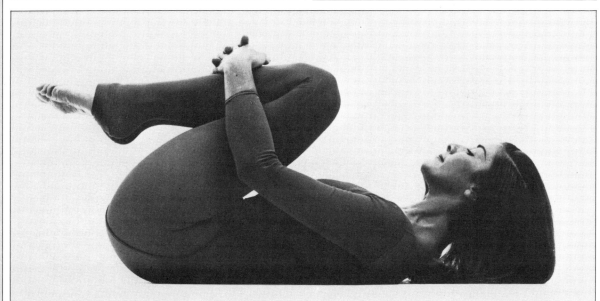

3 Carry your head back as slowly as you can without straining, and when it touches the ground, stay as you are but relax for a few moments before repeating then straighten the legs out in the position of Deep Relaxation again. Do the Coil twice at first and increase gradually to four times.

SECTION 5

BACK PUSH-UP

This movement strengthens the middle of the back and the shoulders, and firms the thighs and buttocks. It is also very effective in eliminating masculine 'pot' belly, and can be used on its own for this purpose.

At the beginning, do not try to raise the back as high as you can. Be content with a moderate raise of a few inches, coming up smoothly and holding your position rock steady for the count. With practice, your raise will go higher and higher.

> **Breathing:**
> Inhale when in starting position.
> Exhale as you raise the back.
> Inhale as the back is lowered.
> Exhale when the back touches the ground.

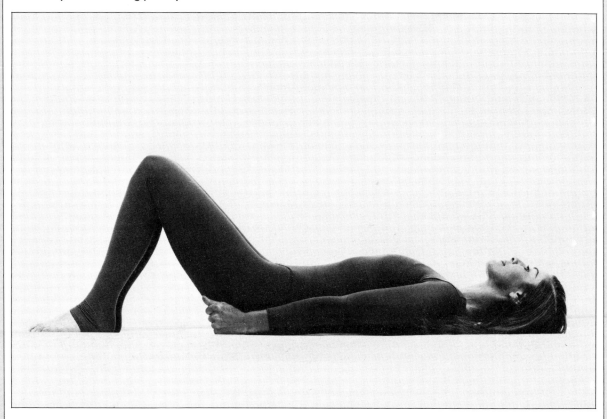

1 Relax for a few moments in the position of Deep Relaxation, and then close the legs and feet and bend the knees, drawing the feet in with the soles of the feet flat on the floor. Keep the knees and feet together and make fists of the hands, thumbs uppermost.

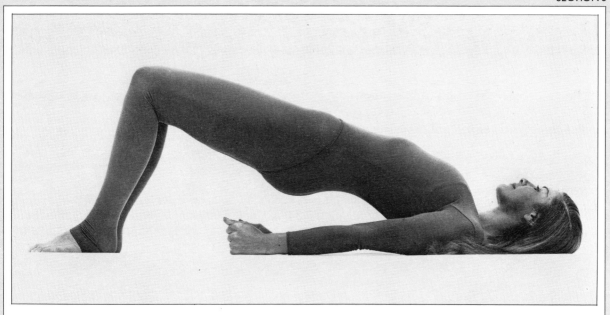

2 Inhale deeply, then push down with the fists and feet, and smoothly raise the body.

Hold the position absolutely still for a count of five.

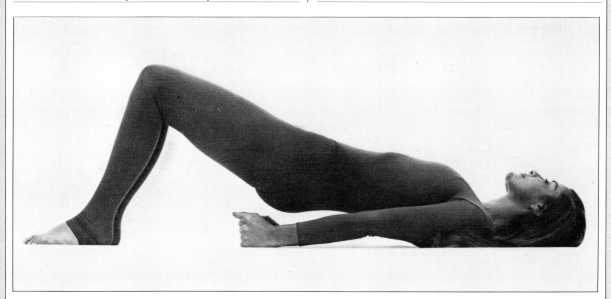

3 Lower the body smoothly and slowly, pressing the knees together to help your control.

When your back touches the ground, let your hands relax palms uppermost but keep the legs and feet as they are.

Rest for a few moments and repeat the movement, before stretching the legs out and going into the position of Deep Relaxation again.

Execute the Push-up twice to begin with, increasing gradually to four times.

FRONT PUSH-UP

This movement stretches and firms the legs and strengthens the toe and ankle joints. It also increases the strength of the arms, wrists and shoulders, and revitalises the entire body with increased blood flow while the trunk is upside down.

When you push up, try to get as pronounced a 'V' shape as you can, coming up high on to the balls of the feet and letting the head hang completely relaxed.

Breathing:
Inhale as for position 2.
Exhale as you hold.
Inhale as the knees are lowered.
Exhale when the knees touch.

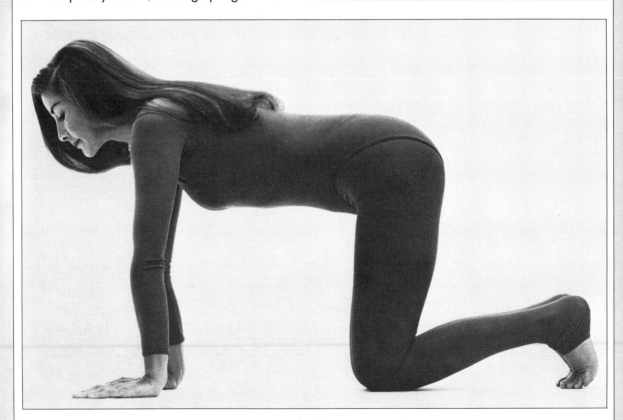

1 Come on to the hands and knees, with the hands directly underneath your shoulders and the knees and feet together. Then tuck your toes under so that you are resting on the balls of the feet.

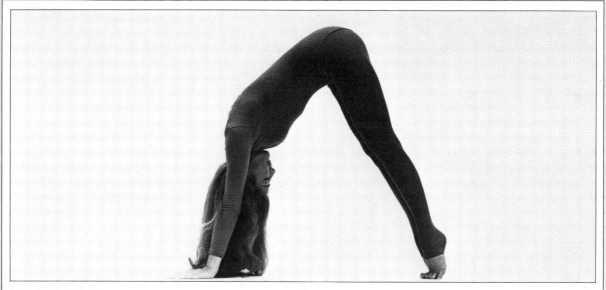

2 Inhale deeply, and push up smoothly. Let your head go completely. Hold your position for a count of five.

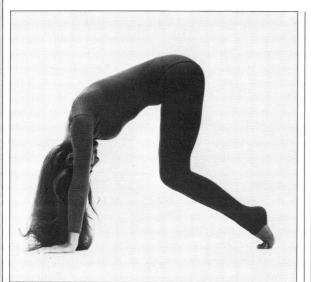

3 Bend the knees slowly, pressing them together to help the control. When they touch the ground, stay as you are, rest for a few moments and then repeat the Push-up movement once again.

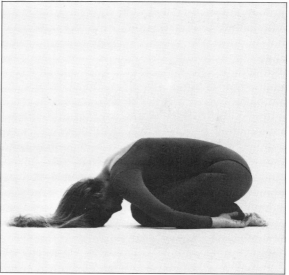

4 After executing the movement twice, come into this relaxation position.

Close your eyes and stay in that position for at least a minute.

Start by executing the Front Push-up twice only, increasing gradually to four times.

SECTION 7

THE LION AND THE JAW LIFT

Now we come to what I consider to be two extremely valuable, if slightly amusing, facial movements.

It has always surprised me that whilst people recognise that muscles in the body will become slack if not used regularly, nobody seems to have realised that exactly the same thing happens with the facial and neck muscles. As we leave childhood, we show less and less spontaneous expression in our faces as we learn, unfortunately, that part of being an adult is to hide or conceal our real emotions. The result of this is that the muscles get used less and less until eventually, if we are not careful, they sag. Regular practice of the Lion and the Jaw Lift will counteract this, by firming the muscles in the face and neck and stimulating increased blood flow in those areas.

As well as the above, these movements also have many other benefits, as you will see, so don't run away with the idea that they are purely cosmetic.

Note: The following four sections are seated movements, and they can be done with the legs crossed as shown, or kneeling and sitting on the heels, or even on a stool or chair if preferred. Whichever position you use, make sure that you sit with your back straight.

THE LION

This is quite a ferocious looking movement and is in fact one of the few aggressive poses in Yoga, so when you do it don't be afraid to be more forceful than with the other postures.

As well as improving the muscle tone in the face and neck, the Lion also strengthens the back, shoulders, arms and hands, and exercises the jaw and tongue. This jaw and tongue movement not only has the effect of strengthening them, but also of stimulating an increased flow of saliva in the mouth that cleanses the taste buds. This means that with regular practice your sense of taste becomes more highly tuned and you will find that you appreciate and enjoy your food much more (see page 15).

When you practise the Lion, as you open the jaw and push the tongue out and down, make a 'Haaaa' roaring sound in your throat as you breathe out, to help you get the correct movement. You may feel slightly ridiculous doing this at first but after two or three times, having begun to feel the benefits, you won't even think about it.

Breathing:
Inhale as for position 2.
Exhale as the tongue comes out and down.
Inhale as the tongue is retracted.
Exhale in resting position 4.

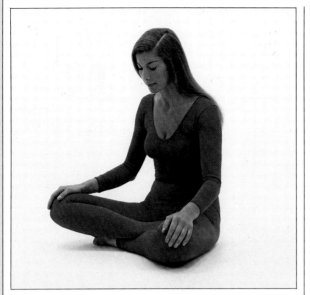

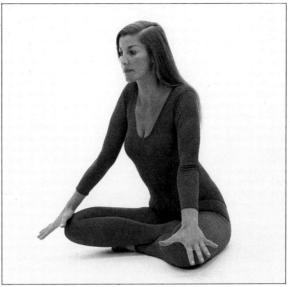

1 Sit with the legs crossed, and the hands resting palms downward on the knees. Relax the head and face.

2 Inhale deeply as you straighten the back, and push down on the knees, spreading the fingers wide.

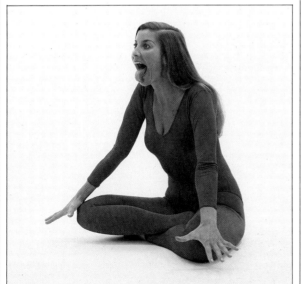

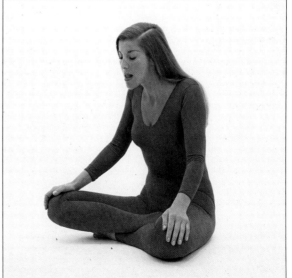

3 Open the eyes as wide as you can, push the jaw open and make the 'Haaaa' sound as you breathe out, pushing the tongue right out and down at the same time. Retain position for a count of five.

4 Retract the tongue, let the back relax, and return to position 1.
  Rest for a few moments, then repeat the Lion a further three times.

THE JAW LIFT

Where the Lion exercises the jaw by opening it wide, the Jaw Lift exercises it the other way, by pushing it up.

The Jaw Lift also firms the chin and eliminates any sagging flesh, which will be good news to anybody with a tendency towards a double chin. This part of the anatomy is particularly difficult to streamline but the Jaw Lift, when done in this position with the head back, really gets to it.

As well as stretching the neck and firming the chin, this movement also increases blood circulation in the face and, as with the Lion, increases the sensitivity of the taste buds and improves cleanliness of the mouth.

Breathing:
Breathe naturally in and out during this movement.

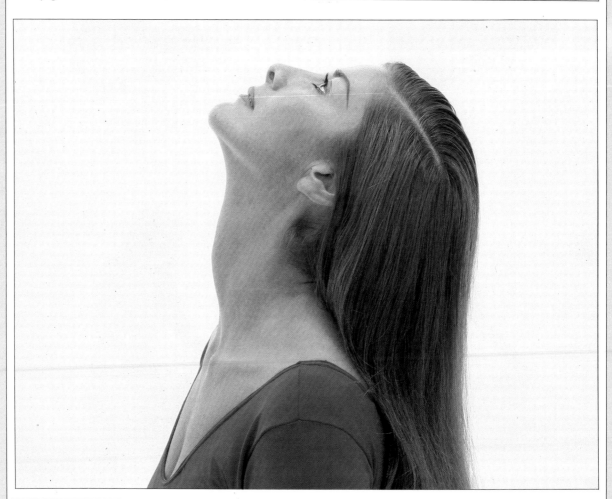

1 Sit straight and gently let the head relax back.

2 Let the bottom part of your jaw drop open – just let it relax.

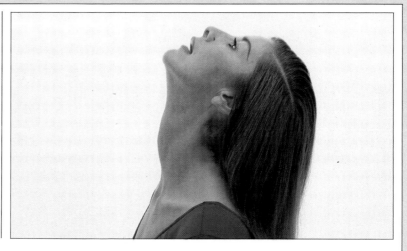

3 Push the bottom part of the jaw forward and out as far as you can and then up as high as you can, bringing your bottom teeth up and over your top teeth and lip.

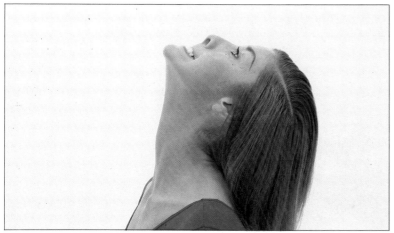

4 Hold the position for only a second or two, then let the jaw drop open again.

Repeat the Jaw Lift a further three times, then close your mouth, let your head relax forward again, close your eyes and rest your face.

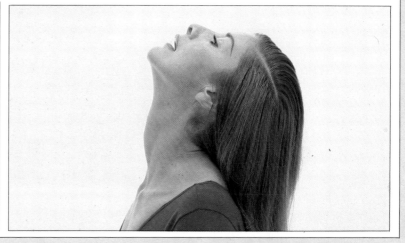

SECTION 8

ALTERNATE NOSTRIL BREATHING

This breathing technique does three things. It clears the mind immediately you begin, establishes deep and even breathing, and relaxes the body. It therefore has all the necessary ingredients to relax you and eliminate tension and anxiety, and it makes this one of the best and most effective natural relaxants around. This means that as well as using the technique in your routine to improve breathing and concentration, you can also use it to great effect at other times during your life, when you are feeling particularly tense or nervous, and need or want to calm yourself down physically, mentally and emotionally (page 14).

This is what actually happens. A breathing rhythm of 4–4–4–4 is established as you breathe in through the left nostril for four, close both nostrils for four, exhale through the right nostril for four and do nothing for the last count of four. You would then immediately repeat breathing in through the right nostril and ending by exhaling through the left nostril. This would complete one revolution.

At first complete two revolutions gradually increasing to four with practice.

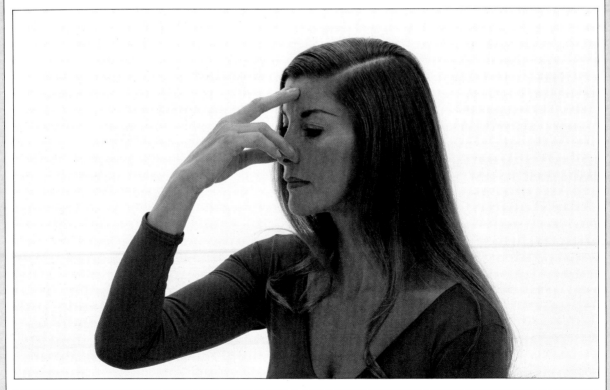

1 Place the first and second fingers of your right hand on your forehead, the third and fourth fingers lightly on your left nostril and your thumb lightly on your right nostril.

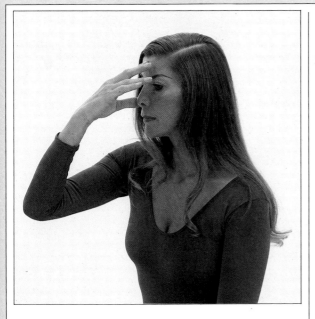

2 Close the right nostril with your thumb and inhale deeply through the left nostril to a count of four.

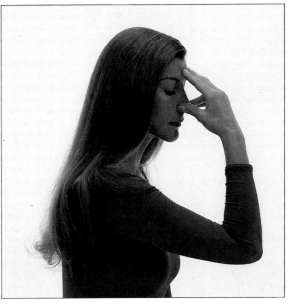

3 Close both nostrils, keeping the breath inside you, for a second count of four.

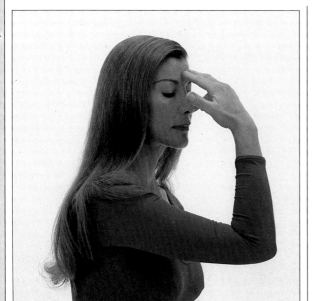

4 Exhale slowly through the right nostril for a third count of four.

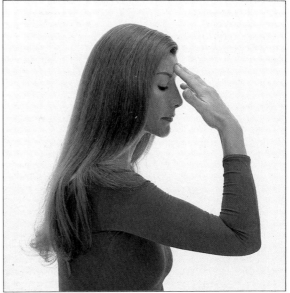

5 Release both nostrils but stay without breath for a fourth count of four. Repeat other way.

SCALP TUGS

'**O**uch!' I hear you say, 'sounds painful'. Well, we're not going to tug the hair right out of the head but, by gripping the roots in a certain way, it is possible to move the scalp and stimulate the blood flow to the hair follicles. This enriches the hair so that it both looks and feels healthier.

As far as men are concerned, loss of hair can be distressing, and although baldness is partially hereditary, many men over the years have reported an improvement in both the quality of their hair and the fact that hair loss seems to occur less frequently.

Breathing:
Breathe naturally during this movement.

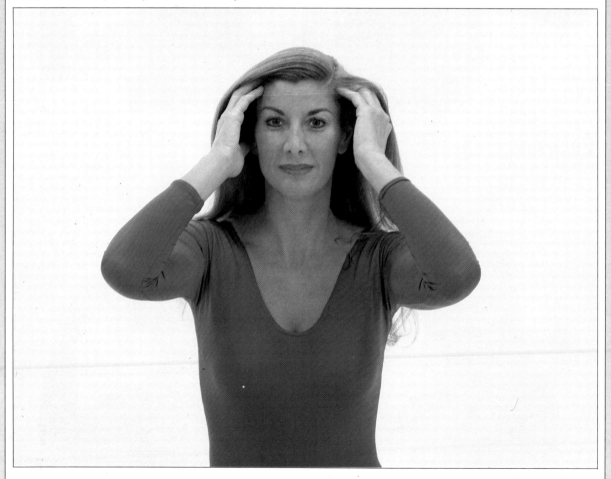

1 Sit comfortably with the back straight and place the fingers at the temples.

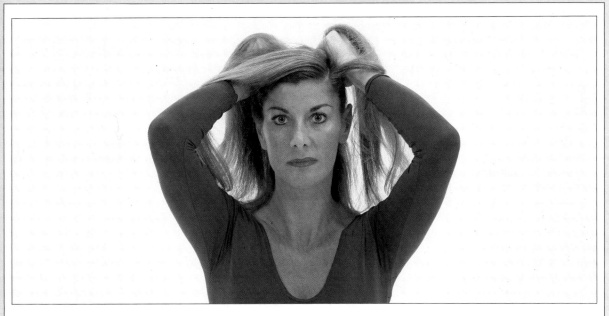

2 Slide the fingertips hard into the scalp towards the crown of the head making tight fists out of the hands gripping the hair as close to the roots as you possibly can.

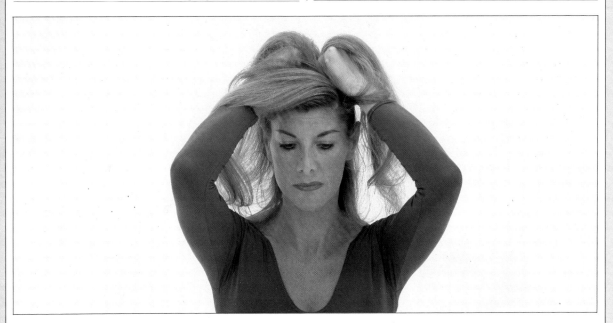

3 Tug gently forwards and backwards with your fists four times, feeling that your scalp is moving just a fraction each time and repeat the movement four times with the hands in the back of the head. Remove your hands and relax them on your knees, close your eyes and rest.

SECTION 9

HEAD ROLL

This movement is not only lovely and relaxing to do but it also gently stretches the neck and throat as well.

It is most beneficial done with the eyes closed, so do this as soon as you have learned it.

As well as being part of your routine, use this movement in your everyday life, to remove stiffness and tension and relax you.

Breathing:
Breathe normally during this movement.

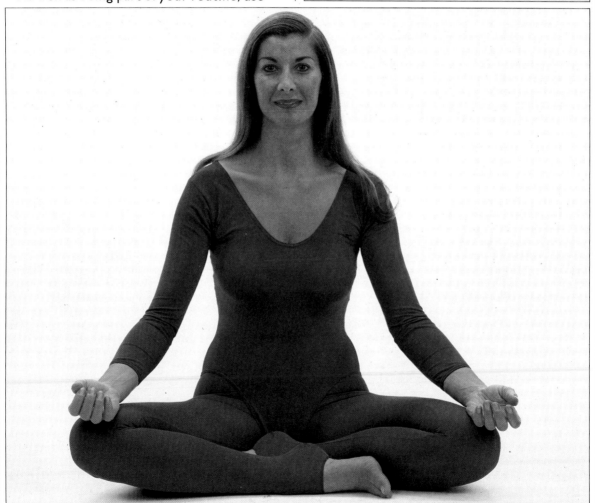

1 Sit comfortably relaxed.

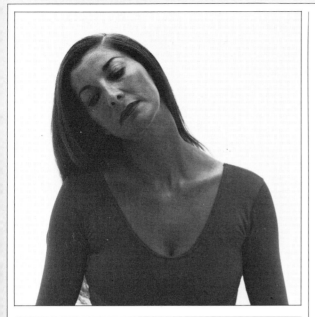

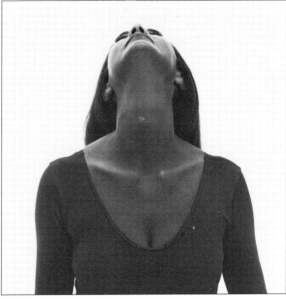

2 Relax the head forward and then gently roll it around to the right. Stop for two or three seconds allowing the weight of the head to take it over to its natural limit.

3 Continue rolling your head to the back, and if your mouth feels it wants to open a little, let it. Stop, letting the head relax back, and pause for two or three seconds.

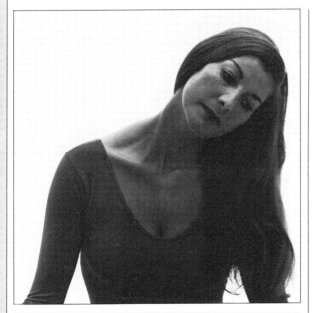

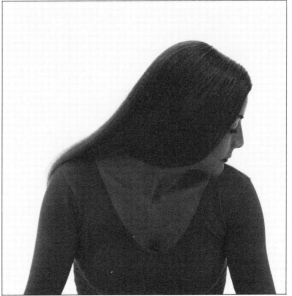

4 Continue slowly to the left allowing the head to rest. Pause for two or three seconds.

5 Turn the head, lower the chin and push the head down as it returns to front. Repeat roll to left.

EYE ROTATIONS

This movement simply exercises the eyes by rotating them in a circle, but making the eyes go to the extreme points of the circle and then focusing them for a second or two.

Breathing:
Breathe naturally during this movement.

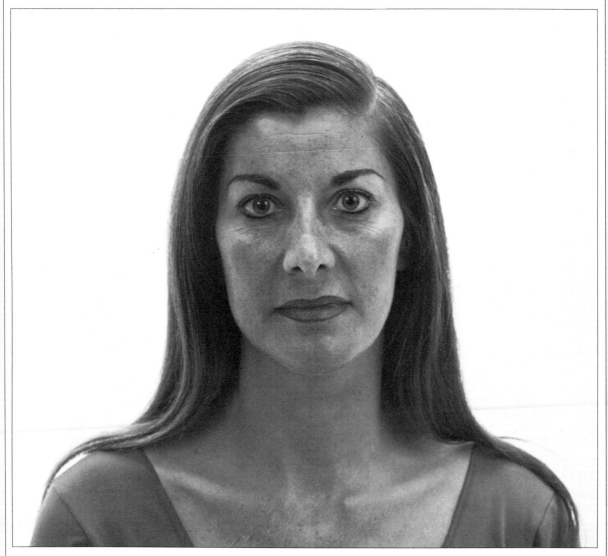

1 Sit with the head erect.

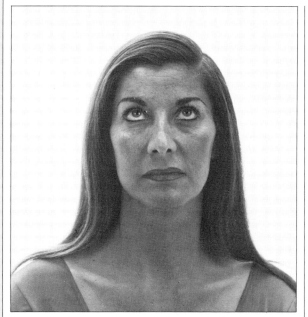

2 Raise your eyes and focus on the ceiling. Pause for a second or two.

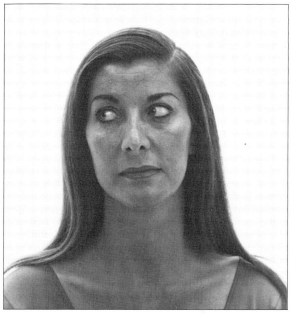

3 Roll your eyes around to your far right and focus for a second or two.

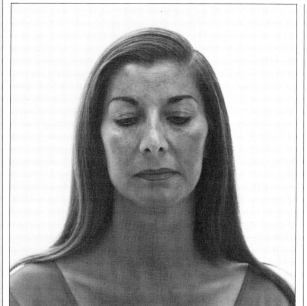

4 Roll your eyes down and look as low as you can. Focus for a second or two.

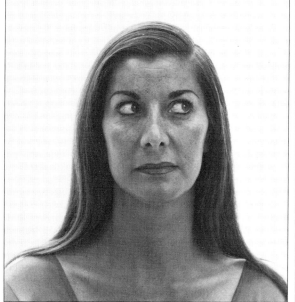

5 Roll your eyes to the left and focus. Return to the ceiling and repeat. Execute twice to left.

FINGER PULLS

The name of this movement is misleading, because it sounds as though only the fingers are exercised. In fact, this movement exercises and strengthens the back, shoulders, upper arms, forearms and finally the finger joints. It also improves breathing and develops the chest.

As you will see, the breathing instructions are integrated with the movement, so try to include them.

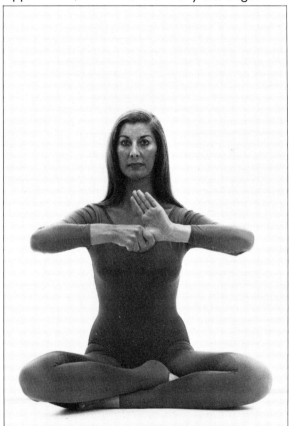

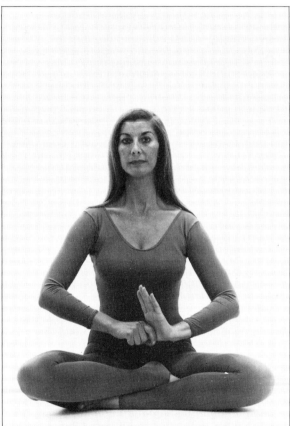

1 Inhale deeply as you grip the thumb, bringing the hands in level with your collar bone and turning the palm of the hand away from you.

2 Hold your breath as you pull hard on the thumb and bring the level of your hands smoothly down to your navel.

Exhale deeply and repeat with the remaining fingers of that hand, then change hands.

After going through all the fingers, let the hands rest on the knees, palms uppermost, fingers relaxed, and rest the head and face.

ELBOW SNAPS

Don't worry, we're not going to snap any bones, but the odd crack may be heard because this movement works out the stiffness in the elbow joints.

The positioning of the hands is extremely important, so really make sure that yours are absolutely correct.

The movement itself actually looks like a punch, but the fists are there to act as shock absorbers as your elbows straighten; so keep them tightly closed.

As you straighten the elbows, try to feel as though you are contracting your elbows in, rather than punching out away from you. In fact, it helps if you imagine that there is a wall less than an arm's length in front of you and you are trying not to hit it as you straighten the arms.

At the beginning, while you learn the positions of the fists, do the movement smoothly, but when you feel you know it sufficiently, straighten the elbows more sharply.

Breathing:
Breathe normally during this movement.

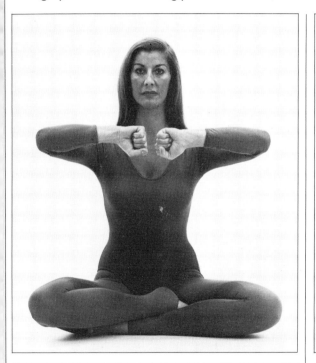

1 Bend the elbows and bring the fists in level with your chest, with the thumbs down towards the floor.

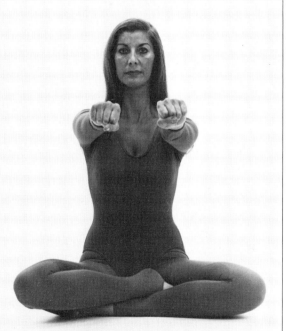

2 Sharply extend your arms, ending with the fists square on, knuckles upwards. Pause only for a fraction of a second, bring the fists into the starting position again and repeat a further five times. Then relax the hands on the knees, palms uppermost, and rest.

SECTION II

KNEE AND THIGH STRETCH

As the name implies, this movement stretches the knees and the thighs, but it gets to an area of the thigh not generally reached in normal exercise – the very top of the inside thigh. Many women will know that this is often regarded as one of the 'problem' areas of the body, and seemingly impossible to slim and firm. However, regular practice of the Knee and Thigh Stretch will do just that.

When you do it, be extremely gentle with yourself. The upper part of the inside thigh is very delicate and not used to being stretched, so do not bounce the knees or jerk, and be prepared for just a little movement at the beginning. Gradually, with gentle practice, your knees will go further and further down towards the floor. (See picture 4)

Breathing:
Inhale when in position 2.
Exhale as knees are pressed down.
Inhale as knees come up again.
Exhale when back in starting position.

1 Bend the knees and bring the soles of the feet together.

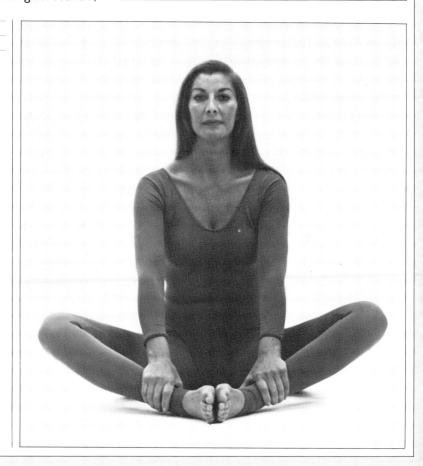

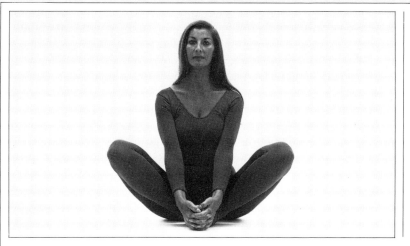

2 Interlock the fingers and loop them around the toes and, using this grip, bring the heels in as close to your body as you can.

3 Keeping the back straight, carefully and smoothly press the knees down towards the floor, stopping the instant you become aware of the stretch along the inside of the upper thigh.

Hold your position for a count of five, then let the knees come up again.

Repeat the movement once more, then stretch both legs out in front, letting them flop relaxed and supporting yourself by putting your hands behind you.

Increase gradually to four times.

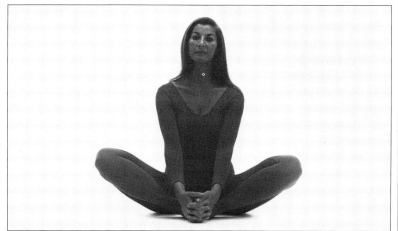

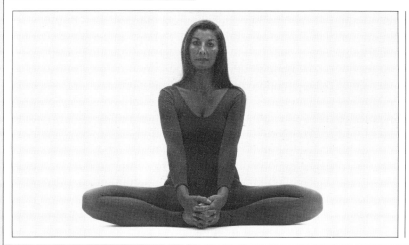

4 In time the knees may touch the ground without forcing.

ANKLE ROTATIONS

This movement works on the toe and ankle joints, getting and keeping them healthy and strong, and it also strengthens the calf muscles.

It is a continuous rotation, but taking the foot to the very extreme positions of the circle.

Breathing:
Breathe naturally during this movement.

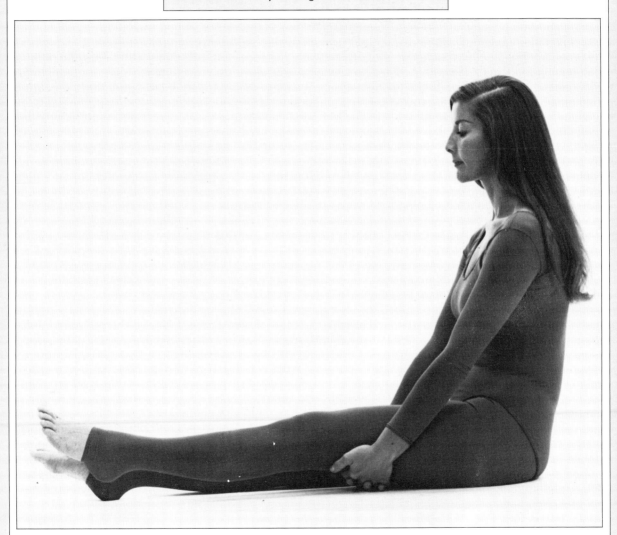

1 Raise the left leg, interlock the fingers and rest the leg on your hands with the knee straight.

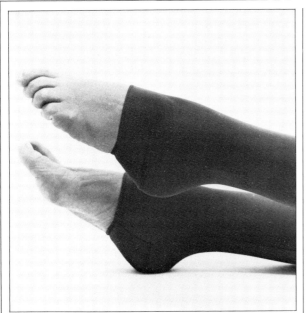

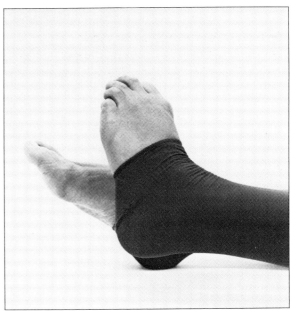

2 Keeping your leg straight and still, point your toes down to the floor.

3 Start to rotate the foot inwards, clenching the toes as you go.

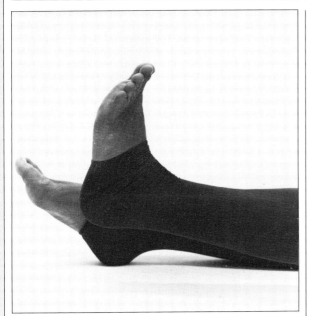

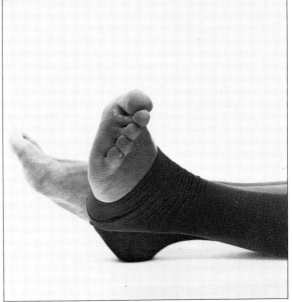

4 Continue to rotate until the foot is straight up, pushing the heel away from you and the toes back towards you.

5 Continue slowly to the outside of your circle, and return to the starting position.
Repeat three times and change legs.

SECTION 12

ALTERNATE LEG PULL

This movement works on each leg individually, not only stretching the backs, but also firming, streamlining and strengthening the thighs and calves. It also gives a wonderful stretch to the lower back and neck, strengthens the arms and shoulders, and loosens the hip joints.

When most people begin to practise this movement, the bent knee is often quite a way off the ground. If this happens to you, don't worry, just let the knee stay where it feels comfortable. As you practise this and the preceding movement regularly, you will find that your knees gradually go down.

Breathing:
Inhale as arms are raised above head (position 2).
Exhale as arms are lowered and leg is gripped.
Inhale as head is pushed back.
Exhale as head relaxes forward.
Inhale as hands slide back up the leg.
Exhale when in starting position again.

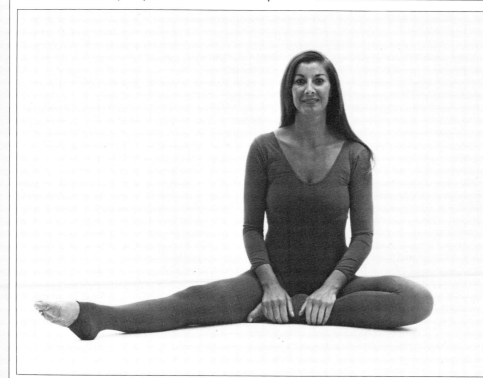

1 Sit with both legs stretched out in front of you. Then bend the left knee and bring the sole of the foot along the inside of the right thigh.

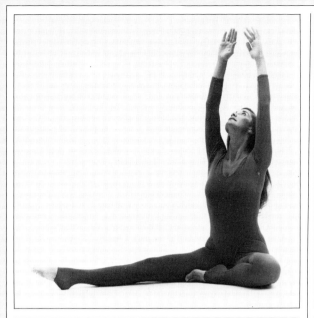

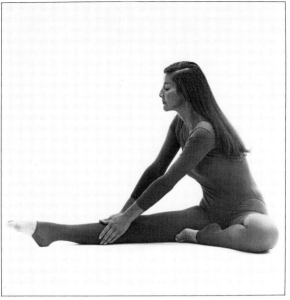

2 Take a deep breath as you raise the arms above your head.

3 Lower your arms and grip your leg just below the knee.

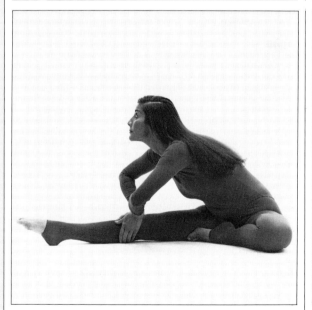

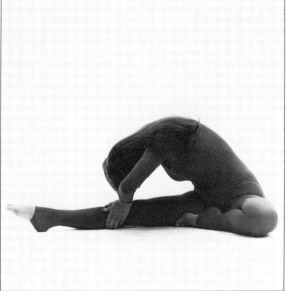

4 Push your head back as far as you can, then pull on the leg, letting your elbows bend out to the sides, so that you feel yourself coming over from the hips, not the waist.

5 Relax the head over and count five in that position. Straighten the elbows and slide the hands back up the legs and then repeat.
Change legs and execute twice on the other side.

59

SLOW MOTION FIRMING

This is a continuous movement with no holding period or pause, and it firms and strengthens virtually the entire length of your body, from head to toe.

As you will see, there is a modified version and the full Slow Motion Firming movement. Begin with the modified version, and allow your strength to build up a bit, especially the abdominal and back muscles. You can then move on to the more advanced version.

MODIFIED SLOW MOTION FIRMING MOVEMENT

The movement simply entails sitting up and then lying down again but it is done in continuous slow motion without using the hands to help you. As you will see, the movement uses a surprising number of muscles.

At the beginning, if you find that your legs and feet come off the ground as you sit up or lie down, it is perfectly permissible to hook your toes underneath a heavy piece of furniture to help. A solid settee or bed that is four to six inches off the ground would be perfect. Prac-

tise like this for a while and then see if the muscles have strengthened enough to sit up and lie down slowly without help.

> **Breathing:**
> Inhale as you sit up (position 2).
> Exhale as arms are lowered.
> Inhale as you roll back down.
> Exhale when head touches.

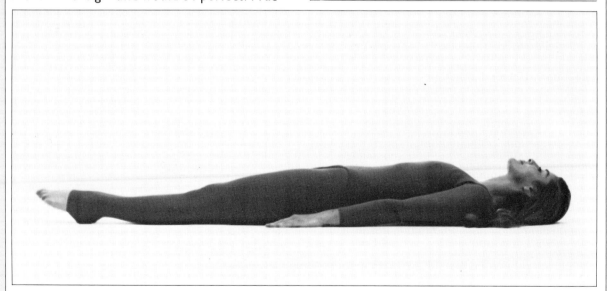

1 Rest for a few moments in the position of Deep Relaxation, then bring the legs and feet together and turn the palms of the hands towards the floor.

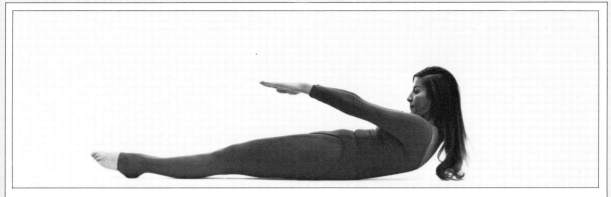

2 Inhale as you reach forward with the arms and hands and sit up smoothly, without bending legs.

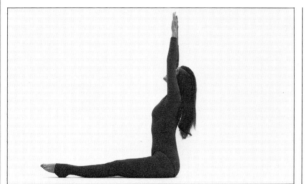

3 Raise the arms above the head and look up.

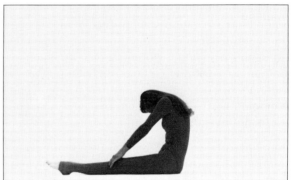

4 Lower the arms and place the hands on top of legs, pushing head down and curving top of back.

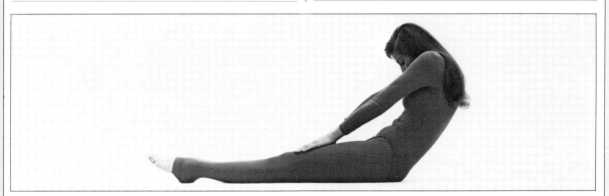

5 Slowly roll back down until you are flat on the floor once more. When the back of your head touches, immediately begin again, keeping the movement continuous and smooth.

Execute the movement twice to begin with, increasing gradually to four times.

FULL SLOW MOTION FIRMING

For the full movement, the knees are first bent in towards your chest, extended, and then lowered slowly. The instant that your legs touch the ground, reach forward with your arms and sit up. Then continue as for the modified version until you are flat on your back again, ready to restart.

Remember the benefit is gained by moving slowly and smoothly all the way through.

Breathing:
Inhale when flat on the floor in starting position
Exhale as knees are bent in towards chest.
Inhale as legs are extended.
Exhale as legs are lowered to floor.
Inhale as you sit up.
Exhale as arms come down onto legs.
Inhale as you roll back down.
Exhale when head touches.

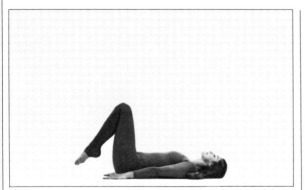

1 Bend both knees in towards your chest.

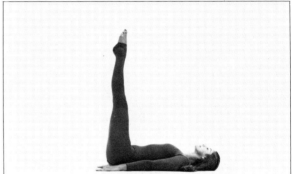

2 Extend the legs into the air.

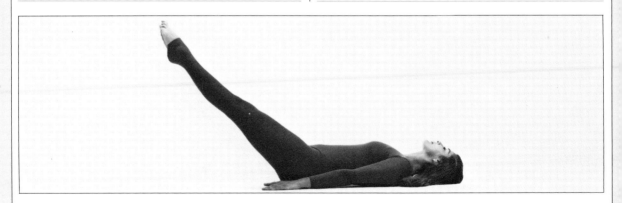

3 Lower the legs slowly.

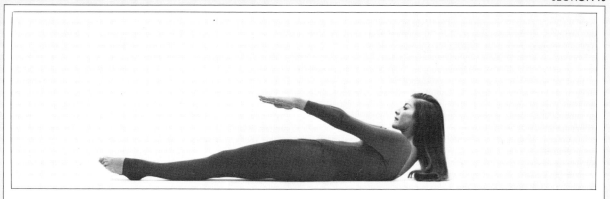

4 When the feet have touched the ground, reach forwards and sit up.

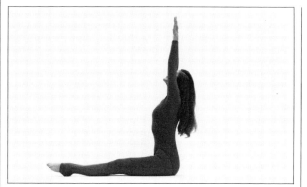

5 Raise the arms above your head.

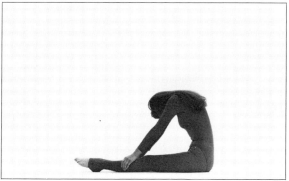

6 Lower the arms and hands onto the legs.

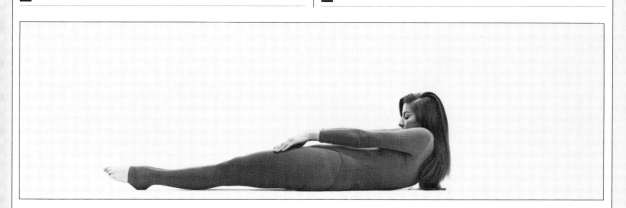

7 Slowly roll back down with the top of the back curved. When your head touches the floor, repeat immediately and then relax in the position of

Deep Relaxation.
  Execute twice at first, increasing gradually to four times.

SECTION 14

SHOULDER STAND

This movement is valuable in so many ways that I felt I had to include it in your routine. It relieves pressure in the legs and feet, improves overall circulation, stimulates the thyroid gland, aiding weight loss, and strengthens the whole body. It also has a revitalising effect on the entire organism.

As you will see, we are going to work towards the completed Shoulder Stand in stages, and there are two modified positions that should be practised first.

A word of caution here:
Many people think that it is quite all right to 'swing' up into the shoulder stand. It is definitely **NOT**. It is extremely dangerous and you could do severe and permanent damage to yourself. The safest and most beneficial way of practising, as with all of these movements, is by exercising complete control every second of the way and doing it slowly and smoothly. The muscles that you need to do this are gradually being strengthened by practising the modified versions, so wait until your body is ready, and don't be tempted to rush or 'swing' prematurely into the more advanced position.

SHOULDER STAND – MODIFIED POSITION 1

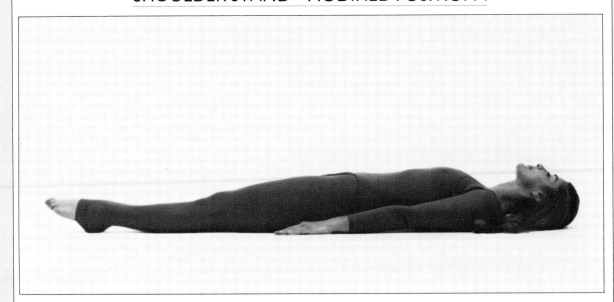

1 Rest for a few moments in the position of Deep Relaxation, then close the legs and feet and turn the palms of the hands towards the floor.

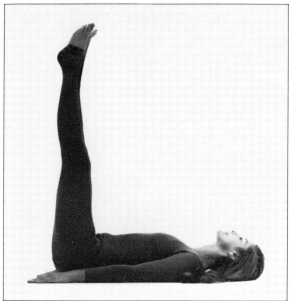

2 Take a deep breath and raise the legs until they are at right angles to the body.

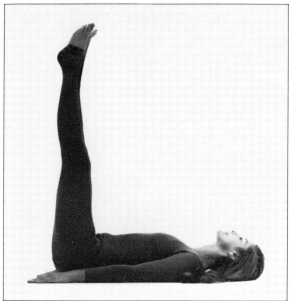

3 Relax the muscles in the legs and feet to allow relief of pressure.

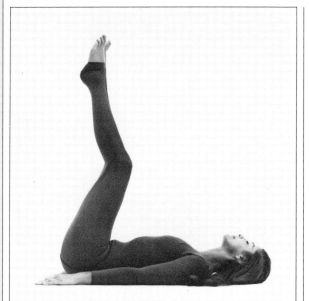

4 You may bend the knees a little if it is more comfortable.

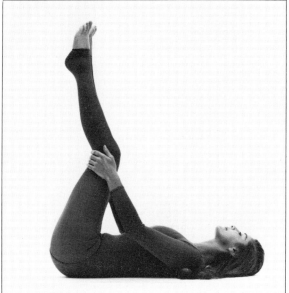

5 Support your legs with your hands if you like. Hold for a count of twenty, then lower the legs slowly. Relax and then repeat.

SHOULDER STAND – MODIFIED POSITION 2

With this second modified position, the body comes off the ground; it is quite a marked progression from the previous position, so try it carefully and gently to see if you are ready.

At the end of the holding period, instead of lowering the legs as before, there is a special rolling out movement that prevents the back from being strained, so take particular note of it and follow the instructions carefully.

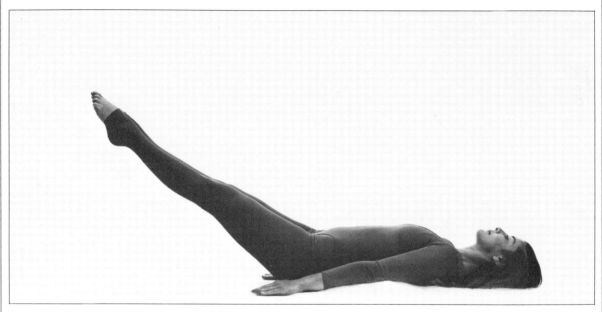

1 Take a deep breath and raise the legs with the knees straight and the feet together.

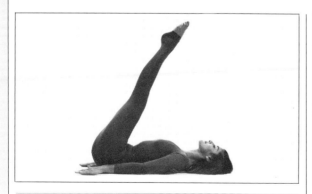

2 As you pass Modified position 1, push down with your hands bringing your legs closer to your head.

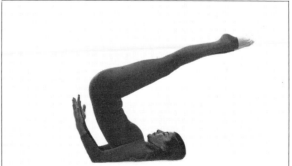

3 Push on the floor with your elbows so that you can bend the arms and bring your hands in to support your back.

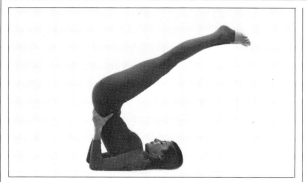

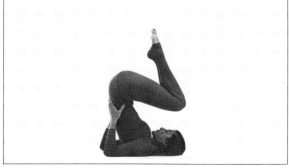

4 Relax the feet muscles but do not bend the knees or you will lose control.
  Count twenty in that position, breathing normally.

5 Carefully bend both knees in towards your chest, without jerking.

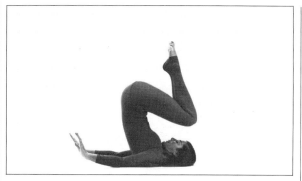

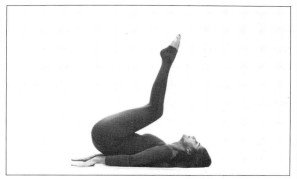

6 Place your hands back on the floor, palms downward. Do this one hand at a time if you feel you have more control that way.

7 Roll out of the position, extending the legs on the way.

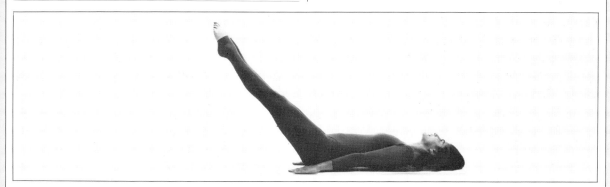

8 Continue lowering the legs slowly, and when they touch the ground, relax once more in the position of Deep Relaxation. Rest for at least 60 seconds. Execute once to begin with and twice only after practising for some time.

COMPLETED SHOULDER STAND

As you practise, your body position will get straighter, and eventually you may be able to attain this position. However, as I have said before, there is no rush, and as long as you are working to your own comfortable and natural limit, you will be benefiting.

Many students in fact never practise this completed position, preferring to stay with Modified position 2. It is more important to feel confident and secure than pushing on to the completed position, no matter what.

1 Completed Shoulder Stand.

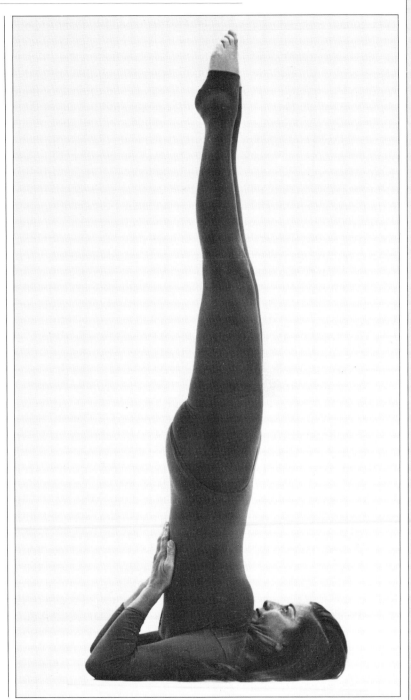

SECTION 15

THE LEG OVER

The final movement in the routine is a wonderful big stretch, that twists and strengthens the centre of the back, and firms and strengthens the legs, buttocks, sides of the torso, shoulders, arms and tummy.

The objective is not to touch the floor as the leg goes over, but to bring the leg over to a comfortable position that can be held still for the count. The weight of your leg during the count is sufficient to bring it over that little bit more to reach your natural limit, and with repeated practice, the leg will go further and further down towards the floor.

It is very important to keep both shoulders 'glued' to the floor as the leg comes across, in order to establish the right twist and stretch through the body, and you can do this by pressing down hard with the palms of the hands.

This is the end of your routine, so after repeating the movement twice on each side really abandon yourself and go into the position of Deep Relaxation for at least five minutes.

Breathing:
Inhale as leg is bent in and extended.
Exhale as leg goes over.
Inhale as leg is carried back.
Exhale as leg is lowered.

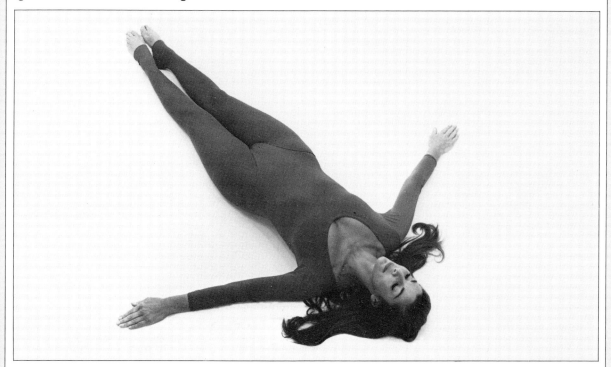

1 After resting in the position of Deep Relaxation for a few moments, close the legs and feet and turn the palms towards the floor. Spread the arms so that they are almost level with the shoulders.

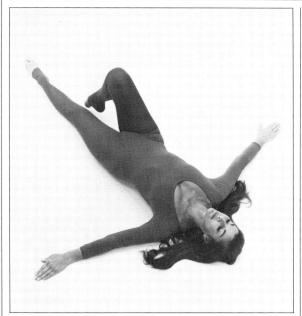

2 Bend the right knee in.

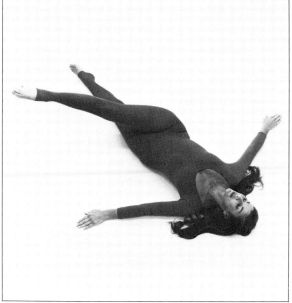

3 Extend the leg.

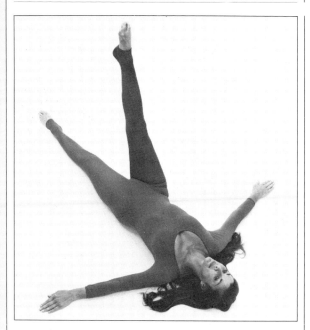

4 Straighten the knee keeping the leg at medium height.

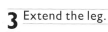

5 Begin to take the leg over to the left.

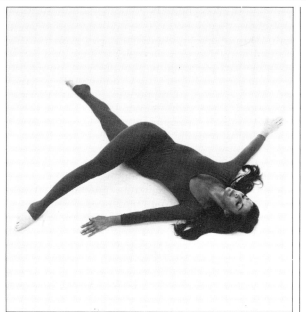

6 Stop in a comfortable position, knees straight, shoulders flat on floor. Hold for a count of five.

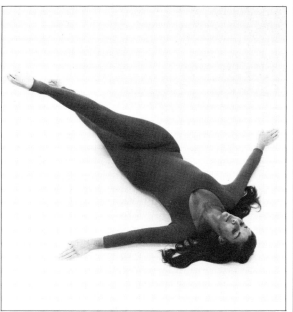

7 Start to carry the leg back . . .

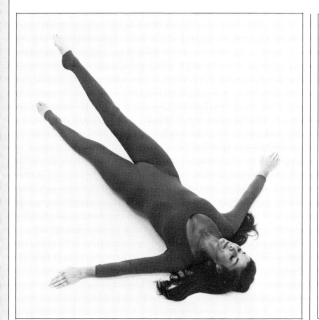

8 . . . until it is straight in front of you again.

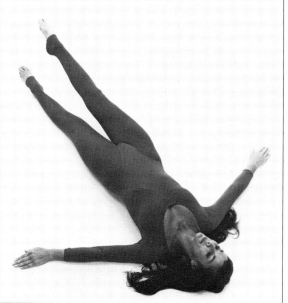

9 Lower the leg slowly and repeat with the left leg. Then repeat once more on both sides.

PRACTICE SECTIONS A-E
ALTERNATIVE MOVEMENTS

The following movements are a little more advanced and may be used in time as alternatives to certain movements in your routine. However, do not consider using them until you have been practising the initial routine for quite some time and feel completely comfortable with it.

When you want to add these movements, use them only one at a time, choosing any one of the five that appeals to you. Once you have integrated it into the routine, practise it for a while and get used to it before adding another.

Remember that these movements are alternatives and not additions to the routine. They have to be substituted for specific existing movements, so that the overall balance and comprehensiveness of the routine is maintained.

Details of which movements to eliminate are set out with each of the following alternatives.

For easy reference, the six pictures on the next page show the movements contained in this practice section and where to find them.

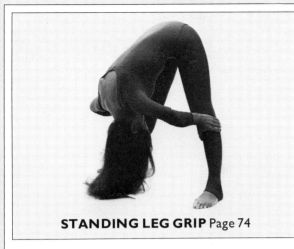

STANDING LEG GRIP Page 74

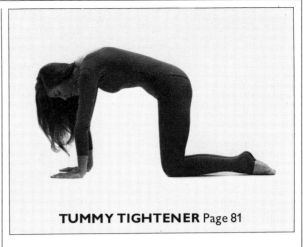

TUMMY TIGHTENER Page 81

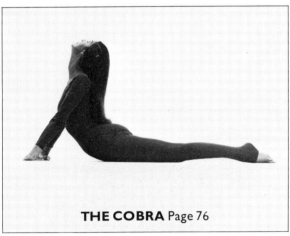

THE COBRA Page 76

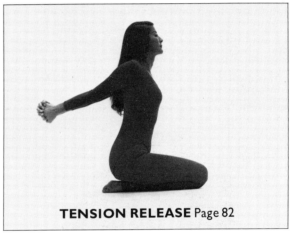

TENSION RELEASE Page 82

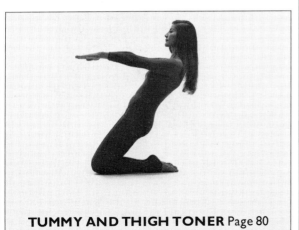

TUMMY AND THIGH TONER Page 80

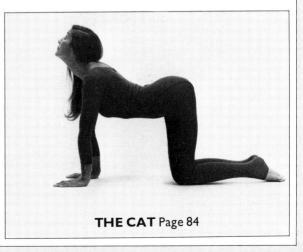

THE CAT Page 84

SECTION A

STANDING LEG GRIP

This is a wonderful movement for stretching the backs of the legs and the lower back, and for strengthening the arms, shoulders and neck. It also improves circulation in the head and face and helps establish good balance and co-ordination.

When you are relaxed over, and about to grip the legs, grip them at whatever level the hands are already hanging. Don't grip any lower down the legs.

Grip the sides of the legs firmly, so that when the arms bend, the elbows go out to the sides.

> **Breathing:**
> Inhale as in picture 2.
> Exhale as head goes over (Picture 4).
> Inhale as arms are straightened again.
> Exhale as head is lifted a little.

Slot the Leg Grip into the routine after the Triangle, page 30, executing it after relaxing over at the end in the Refresher position. You can then carry on afterwards, slowly uncoiling the back as shown.

(Exchange the Standing Leg Grip for the Front Push-up on page 38.)

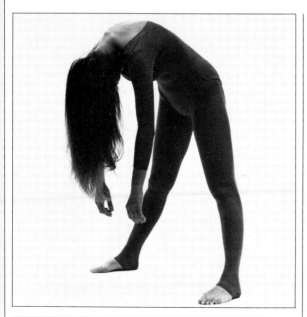

1 Relax the body over to its natural limit.

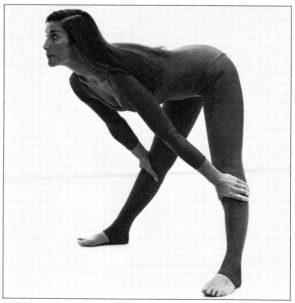

2 Grip the legs and raise the face as much as you can.

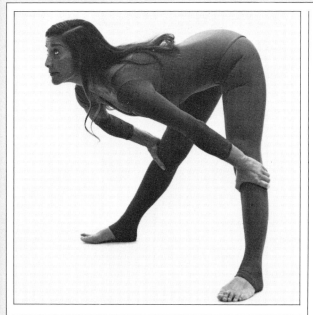

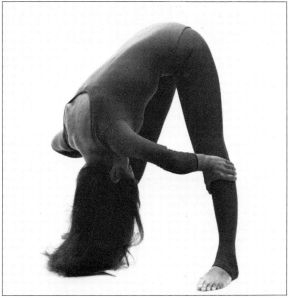

3 Keeping face raised, inhale deeply and pull on the legs letting elbows bend to the side, so your body comes over from hips, not waist.

4 Try to get your chin as close to your chest as you can comfortably and count five in that position.

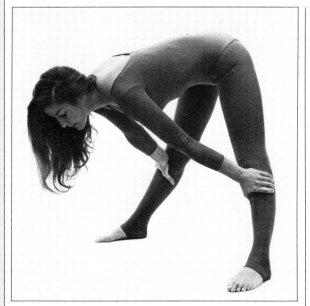

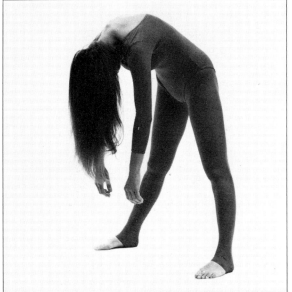

5 Straighten the elbows and raise the head a fraction, rest for a few moments and repeat.

6 After doing the Leg Grip twice, let your body relax over and then slowly uncoil. Gradually increase to four times with practice.

SECTION B

THE COBRA

This movement arches the back not unlike the shape that a Cobra makes, and hence its name. As well as strengthening and increasing the suppleness of the back, it also strengthens the arms, shoulders, wrists and neck.

It is not a push-up, and the back is arched from the moment the head is raised off the ground.

The objective is not to get the elbows straight but to come to a comfortable position with the head right back and the shoulders back and down, and to hold that position still for the count. In time, as your back strengthens, your elbows will straighten.

> **Breathing:**
> Breathe naturally in and out during this movement.

(Exchange the Cobra for the Fish movement, page 32, then you can roll over on to your back afterwards and continue the routine with the Coil.)

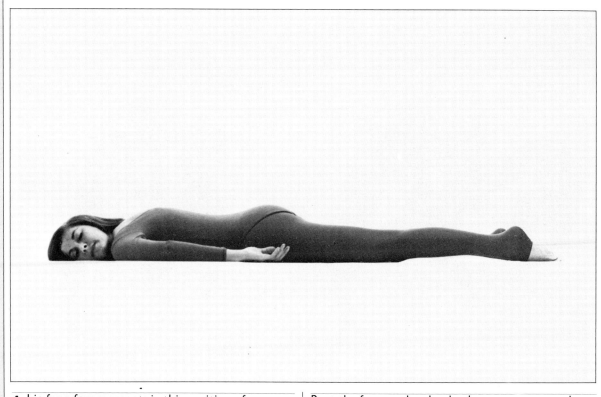

1 Lie for a few moments in this position of relaxation.

Rest the face on the cheek, close your eyes, and relax the legs, feet, arms and hands.

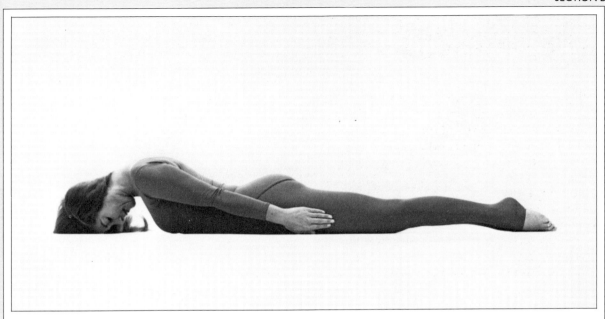

2 Close the legs and feet, bring the hands into your sides, and place the forehead on the ground as high on to your hairline as possible.

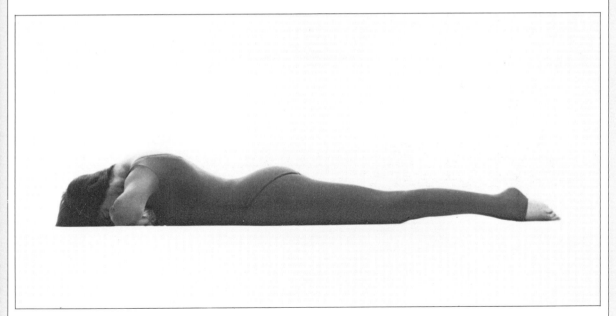

3 Bring your hands in to rest palms downward underneath your shoulders, fingers pointing in towards each other, the elbows out to the sides. Try to get the elbows flat on the floor if you can.

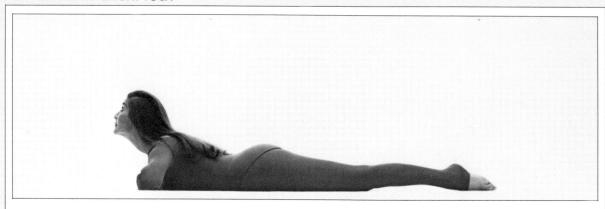

4 Start to raise the head slowly, looking at the ceiling.

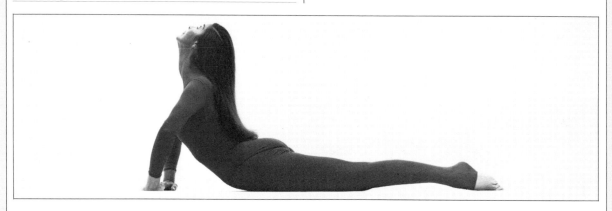

5 Keeping the head right back, slowly push down with the hands.

Stop in a comfortable position and hold for the count of five.

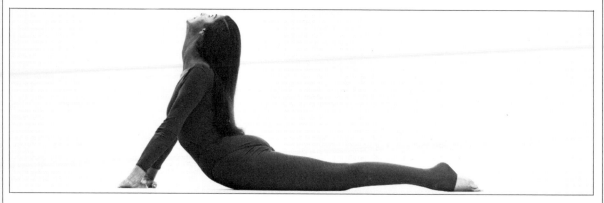

6 In time you may be able to get the elbows completely straight like this without forcing.

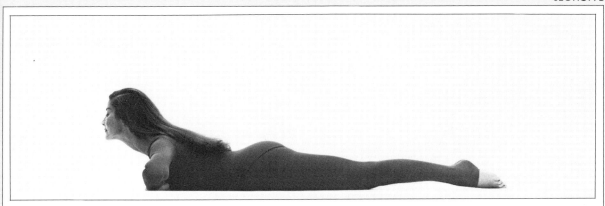

7 Let the elbows bend slowly and bring the body down.

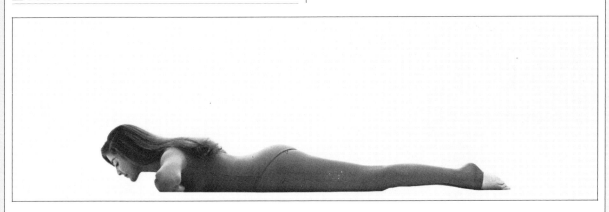

8 Bring the head to the floor again.

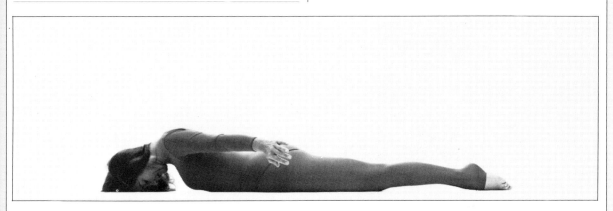

9 Take the arms around to the sides, then relax as in position 1 for a few moments.

Repeat entire movement once more, and then relax again.

SECTION C

TUMMY AND THIGH TONER

This extremely simple-looking movement does what it says; it tones and flattens the tummy and firms the thighs.

The movement works quite strongly on the muscles, and you need only lean back a few inches to have the desired firming effect. However, it is essential that you lean back with the body in a perfectly straight line from the shoulder to the knee (see picture 2). Don't allow your bottom to drop or your back to arch.

Breathing:
Inhale when in upright position.
Exhale as you lean back.
Inhale as you straighten up.
Exhale as you pause before repeating.

(Swop the Tummy and Thigh Toner and the Tummy Tightener, for the Back Push-up, page 36 and the Front Push-up, page 38.)

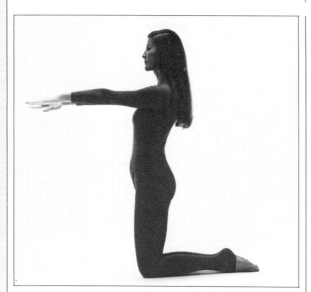

1 Kneel with the back straight, and the knees and feet together, and raise your arms until they are level with the shoulders, palms towards the floor.

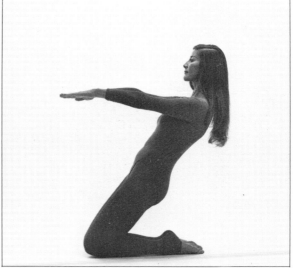

2 Take a deep breath and lean back just a few inches, keeping the back straight. As soon as you become aware of the stretch along the thighs and the tummy, stop and hold your position for a second or two only, then smoothly return to the upright position.

Repeat three more times and then relax by sitting back on to the heels, bringing the forehead down on to the floor, and relaxing the arms, hands and shoulders. (See page 39.)

TUMMY TIGHTENER

This contracting movement tightens the muscles in the whole abdominal and stomach area, having a flattening and firming effect.

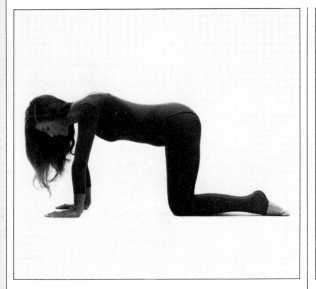

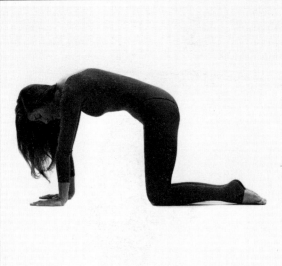

1 Come on to the hands and knees, with the hands directly underneath the shoulders and the knees and feet a few inches apart.

2 Exhale through the nose and contract the abdominal muscles in and up underneath the rib cage. Hold for a count of five.

Then relax the stomach muscles, rest and breathe normally for a few moments.

Repeat the contracting movement three more times, then relax by sitting back onto the heels. (See page 39.)

TENSION RELEASE

This movement relieves the tension that accumulates in the top of the back, and can sometimes cause quite severe pain. If this situation occurs in your daily life, then use the Tension Release to relieve it.

It can be done standing, kneeling or sitting, so choose the position that suits you best depending on your surroundings at the time. Don't forget to loosen the clothing around your neck and waist.

When integrating the movement into the routine, use either the kneeling position shown, or sit cross-legged on the floor, or on a stool, making sure that your back is straight.

As well as removing tension, this movement also strengthens the arms, shoulders and back, and develops the chest. It also slims the diaphragm and waist.

The positioning of fingers, hands, arms and shoulders is extremely important if you are to get maximum benefit from the movement, so please take note of every little detail before you start.

Breathing:
Inhale as arms come round (picture 2).
Exhale as hands are interlinked behind you (picture 3).
Inhale as shoulder rotation begins.
Exhale as shoulder rotation ends.
Inhale as arms are raised.
Exhale as arms are lowered.

(Exchange the Tension Release movement for the Head Roll and Eye Rotation movements pages 48, 50.)

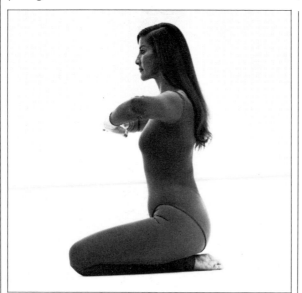

1 Kneel with the seat on the heels and the back straight, and bring the hands in level with the chest, palms downward.

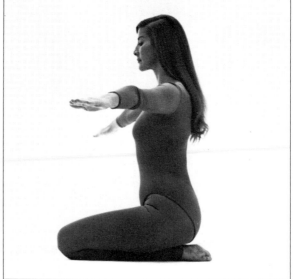

2 Take the arms around at shoulder level.

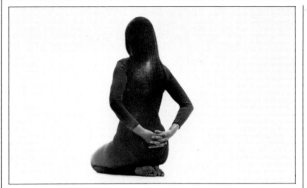

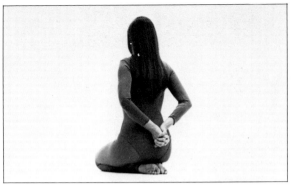

3 Bring the hands in behind you, bending the elbows and interlocking the fingers.

4 Now press the palms of the hands together.

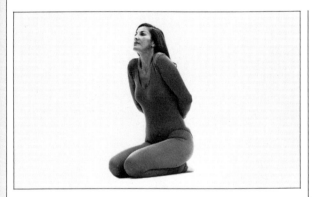

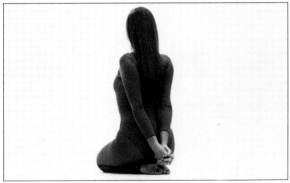

5 Rotate the shoulders forwards and up and then over, back and down.

6 Straighten the elbows, keeping the palms together.

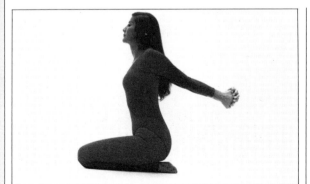

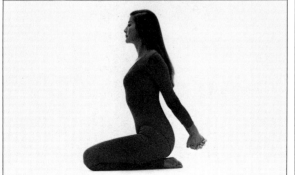

7 Raise the arms just a few inches to a position that you can hold still for a count of five.
Note: Your arms will go higher with practice.

8 Lower the arms smoothly then place the hands in the lap and relax the head and shoulders forward.

THE CAT

This movement really mimics a cat when it is arching and then hollowing its back, and it builds tremendous strength and suppleness in the spine. It also firms and slims the buttocks, waist, hips, thighs, shoulders and upper arms.

Try to move slowly and smoothly as you go from the arched position to the hollowed back position, stopping only for the holding periods.

(Exchange the Cat movement for both the Fish and Coil movements page 32 and page 34.)

Breathing:
Breathe naturally during this movement.

Note: The pictures for this movement have been set out so that it is easier to see the back movement. Read down the page rather than across and follow the numbered captions.

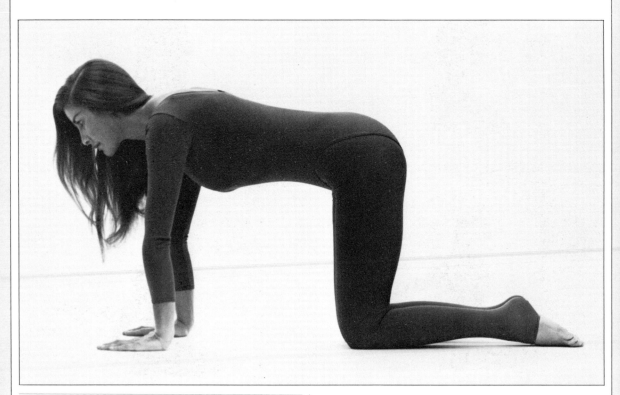

1 Come on to the hands and knees, with the hands directly underneath the shoulders, and the knees and feet a few inches apart.

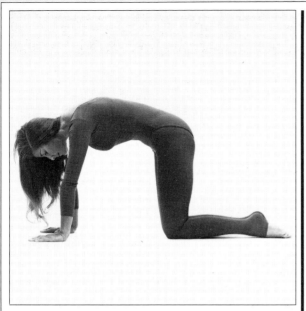

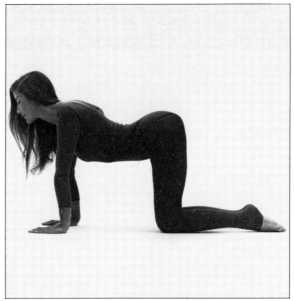

2 Start to arch the back upwards, pushing the pelvis forward a little and letting the head relax forwards.

4 Let the back sink down slowly, pushing the bottom right up and out, really gripping the buttock muscles.

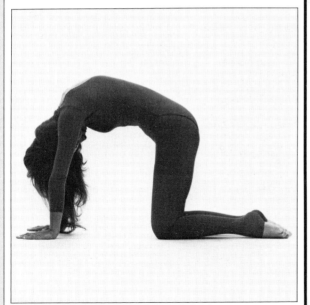

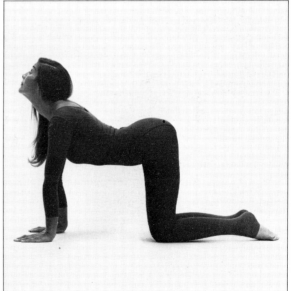

3 Push the pelvis forward even more and get the chin as close to the chest as is comfortable. Count five in that position.

5 With elbows straight, raise the face to the ceiling. Hold for five and repeat movement three more times before relaxing forward, see page 39.

SHORTENED PRACTICE ROUTINES

These routines lasting twenty, thirty and forty minutes, though shortened, have been very carefully compiled so that they still get to every part of the body. Take at least the time specified for each routine as it is the mini- mum required for you to benefit physically and mentally. In particular, do not reduce the relaxation periods at the beginning and end of the routine to less than four minutes.

ROUTINES FOR TWENTY MINUTES

ROUTINES FOR THIRTY MINUTES

ROUTINES FOR FORTY MINUTES

GLOSSARY

GLOSSARY OF MOVEMENTS AND TECHNIQUES

Whilst all of these movements and techniques work perfectly as part of the routine, they can also be extremely valuable when performed and practised entirely on their own.

Many of today's common conditions and ailments can be greatly helped by the practice of specific movements, and I have recommended here the movements and techniques which bring maximum relief and benefit for some of these.

THE POSITION OF DEEP RELAXATION (PAGE 22)

In this position, literally all the muscles in the body are able to relax completely. The breathing apparatus is not restricted allowing the deep and even breathing necessary for complete relaxation.

Use specifically for the following:

1 To relax and unwind completely at any time of the day.
2 To improve your quality of sleep at night.

Note: Use with the mind clearing technique on pages 22, 23 for maximum effect.

THE COMPLETE BREATH (PAGE 24)

This movement combines the raising and lowering of the arms with deep breathing, promoting an increased intake of air and oxygen to the lungs. It also gently stretches the sides, back, arms and shoulders.

Use specifically for the following:

1 To improve breathing generally.
2 To help asthmatic and bronchial disorders.
3 To alleviate fatigue.
4 To improve balance and co-ordination.
5 To wake the system up gently after relaxing or sleeping.

THE STANDING STRETCH (PAGE 26)

This is a completely comprehensive stretch, taking in the arms, legs, sides, shoulders and neck. As well as stretching these areas, the movement also strengthens them.

Use specifically for the following:

1 To stretch and strengthen the entire body.
2 To improve stability and balance of the body.
3 To slim the torso.
4 To increase the suppleness of the spine.

THE REFRESHER (PAGE 28)

This movement relaxes, refreshes and strengthens the body. It has a particularly dramatic effect on the suppleness and strength of the spine.

Use specifically for the following:

1 To relax the mind and body when feeling particularly tense.
2 To ease stiffness in the back or neck.
3 To improve skin disorders, especially in the face.
4 To eliminate fatigue and to improve circulation.
5 To increase strength and suppleness of the joints and muscles in the back.

THE TRIANGLE (PAGE 30)

This movement stretches the sides of the body and firms and slims the arms, shoulders, waist and hips. It also strengthens the back and leg muscles.

Use specifically for the following:

1 To slim the torso.
2 To improve stability and co-ordination.
3 To develop the chest area.
4 To strengthen the back, legs, arms and shoulders.

THE FISH (PAGE 32)

A lovely gentle arching movement for the back that introduces and then maintains suppleness and strength throughout the spine. It also strengthens the shoulders, arms and neck and develops the chest area.

Use specifically for the following:

1 To develop the chest and bust.
2 To increase strength in the shoulders and arms.
3 To eliminate stiffness and tension in the back and neck.
4 To improve the complexion.
5 To increase suppleness in the back.
6 To induce relaxation.

THE COIL (PAGE 34)

With this movement, the spine is stretched from the base right to the tip, not only making it more supple, but also strengthening it. The Coil also slims and firms the buttock muscles, shoulders and arms, and strengthens the neck.

Use it specifically for the following:

1 To stretch, strengthen and then relax the neck muscles.

2 To eliminate flab from the buttocks.
3 To eliminate stiffness from the shoulders.
4 To increase mobility in the spine.
5 To relieve flatulence.

THE BACK PUSH-UP (PAGE 36)

This movement strengthens the centre of the back and firms and strengthens the calves, thighs, buttocks, shoulders and arms. It also works on the muscles around the diaphragm to tighten them.

Use specifically for the following:

1 To spot reduce the 'gut' area. (This is especially effective for men.)
2 To trim and firm the backs of the thighs and buttocks.
3 To develop the shoulder and arm muscles.

THE FRONT PUSH-UP (PAGE 38)

This movement stretches the backs of the legs and firms the calves and the thighs. It also strengthens the toes, ankles, shoulders, arms and wrists, and works on the back muscles increasing suppleness.

Use specifically for the following:

1 To streamline the legs.
2 To improve the strength of the toe, ankle and wrist joints.
3 To improve the complexion.
4 To improve circulation throughout the entire body.

THE LION (PAGE 40)

A wonderful movement for improving the muscle tone in the face. It also exercises and strengthens the jaw and the tongue and promotes increased sensitivity of the taste buds. It also strengthens the back, arms and fingers and loosens the hip joints.

Use The Lion specifically for the following:

1 To firm the facial muscles.
2 To work and subsequently strengthen the jaw and tongue.
3 To get the body used to sitting in the cross-legged position comfortably.

THE JAW LIFT (PAGE 42)

This movement stretches the chin and neck and works on the lower jaw.

Use specifically for:

1 Eliminating a double chin or a suspected tendency towards this.
2 To stretch the neck and throat, firming and streamlining them.
3 To improve the strength of the lower jaw.
4 To increase circulation in the neck and face improving muscle tone.
5 To cleanse the taste buds increasing sensitivity and appreciation of food.

ALTERNATE NOSTRIL BREATHING (PAGE 44)

This technique is a natural tranquilliser. It provides the three ingredients necessary to remove tension and anxiety and promote a state of quiet calm relaxation. The three ingredients are a clear mind, even regular breathing and a relaxed body.

Use specifically for the following:

1 To eliminate insomnia.
2 To alleviate headache and migraine.
3 To improve breathing generally.
4 To help alleviate asthmatic and bronchial conditions.
5 To relieve sinusitis.
6 To relax and eliminate anxiety and tension at any time.
7 To relieve nasal catarrh.
8 To promote deep and relaxed sleep.

9 To relieve fatigue.
10 To help eliminate nervous conditions and phobias such as: Agoraphobia, claustrophobia, fear of flying and lifts etc. Stuttering, nail biting, nausea.

SCALP TUGS (PAGE 46)

This movement improves circulation under the scalp to feed the hair follicles, improving both the condition and appearance of the hair.

Use specifically for the following:

1 To help prevent falling and thinning hair.
2 To promote good circulation in the scalp.

THE HEAD ROLL (PAGE 48)

This movement gently stretches the sides, back and front of the neck and works out stiffness and tension from the top of the back and neck.

Use specifically for the following:

1 To stretch, strengthen and then relax all the neck muscles.
2 To relax both the mind and the body whenever necessary.
3 To relieve tension in the top of the back and shoulders.
4 To relieve general fatigue.

EYE ROTATIONS (PAGE 50)

This subtle movement exercises the eyes.

Use specifically to help alleviate eye strain.

FINGER PULLS (PAGE 52)

This movement strengthens the finger joints, forearms, upper arms, shoulders and back. It also improves the breathing generally and develops the chest area.

Use specifically for the following:

1 To increase strength and agility in the fingers, wrists and arms.
2 To expand the lungs increasing air and oxygen intake.
3 To build up the chest or bust.
4 To increase strength in the upper back and shoulders.

ELBOW SNAPS (PAGE 53)

This movement works to promote strong and healthy elbow joints. It also strengthens the shoulders, arms and hands.

THE KNEE AND THIGH STRETCH (PAGE 54)

This movement stretches, firms and slims the upper and inner thigh, and it also strengthens the back, shoulders, arms and knees.

Use specifically for the following:

1 To slim and firm the inside of the upper thigh.
2 To loosen the hip joints and make them more flexible.
3 To help achieve the cross-legged position with comfort.
4 To maintain strength in the back.

ANKLE ROTATIONS (PAGE 56)

This movement works on the toe and ankle joints. It also strengthens the calf muscles.

Use specifically for the following:

1 To eliminate stiffness of the toes and ankles.
2 To slim the ankles.
3 To improve circulation in the lower legs and the feet.
4 To relieve the pressure caused by prolonged wearing of fashion shoes, especially for women, and allow the feet muscles to relax completely.

ALTERNATE LEG PULLS (PAGE 58)

This stretches the backs of the legs and slims, firms and tightens the thighs and the calves. It also strengthens the lower back, shoulders and arms and loosens the hip joints.

Use specifically for the following:

1 To trim and firm the legs.
2 To stretch the hamstring muscles at the backs of the legs.
3 To increase strength and mobility in the back and especially the lower back.
4 To stretch and then relax the neck.
5 To increase the comfort of the cross-legged seated position.

SLOW MOTION FIRMING (PAGE 60)

This continuous motion technique stretches, strengthens and firms the entire body.

Use specifically for the following:

1 To loose weight and firm the waist, hips, stomach, buttocks, upper arms, shoulders and legs.

THE SHOULDER STAND
(First Position) (PAGE 64)

This modified position inverts the legs and feet in order to relieve pressure. It also strengthens the legs, feet and back.

Use specifically for the following:

1 Relief of tired aching legs and feet.
2 A tendency towards varicose veins.
3 To counteract the stress and strain caused by spending long periods on the feet.
4 Simply to relax and refresh the body.

THE SHOULDER STAND
(Second Position) (PAGE 66)

This movement builds great strength in the back. It also improves the muscle tone in the legs, feet, shoulders and arms and strengthens the abdominal and stomach areas.

Use specifically for the following:

1 To strengthen and refresh the entire body.
2 To relieve pressure from the legs and feet.
3 To stimulate the thyroid gland promoting weight loss and re-distribution.
4 To increase muscle control throughout the body, improving co-ordination and physical stability.
5 To eliminate general fatigue.
6 To improve circulation throughout the body.

THE FULL SHOULDER STAND (PAGE 68)

The completed position refreshes and revitalises the body by reversing the effects of gravity. It also has the benefits of the second Modified position of the shoulder stand.
   Do not attempt it until all of the muscles have built up sufficient strength to enable you to perform the movement with absolute smoothness and control.

THE LEG OVER (PAGE 69)

This movement twists and stretches the body improving the strength of the centre of the back, legs, feet, shoulders and arms. It also slims the torso, hips, waist, stomach and buttocks.

Use specifically for the following:

1 To improve strength in the centre of the back and legs.
2 To streamline the body.
3 To achieve a really comprehensive head to toe stretch.
4 To tone up the stomach and abdominal muscles.
5 To firm the thighs and the buttocks.
6 To slim the waist.

THE STANDING LEG GRIP (PAGE 74)

This movement stretches the back, especially the base of the back, to introduce and then maintain strength and suppleness. It also stretches the backs of the legs and firms the calf and thigh muscles. The shoulders, arms and neck muscles are also strengthened.

Use specifically for the following:

1 To improve the complexion as a result of the increased blood flow into the head and face.
2 To increase balance and stability.
3 To stretch the lower back, increasing the strength of this vulnerable area.
4 To revitalise and refresh the body by inverting it.
5 To improve the circulation generally.

THE COBRA (PAGE 76)

This movement works on the back joints and muscles, increasing strength and suppleness throughout the spine. It also builds the muscles of the shoulders and arms and stretches the neck and throat.

Use specifically for the following:

1 To improve the strength of the arms and shoulders.
2 To eliminate stiffness and tension from the top of the back and the neck.
3 To develop the chest and bust areas.

THE TUMMY AND THIGH TONER (PAGE 80)

This tightens and firms the tummy, abdominal area and the thighs, and it also builds strength into the back, arms and shoulders.

Use specifically for the following:

1 To lose excess inches on the tummy and the thighs.
2 To firm the tummy, stomach and abdominal areas.

THE TUMMY TIGHTENER (PAGE 81)

This technique flattens the tummy and firms and tightens the stomach muscles.

Use specifically for the following:

1 To help alleviate constipation and flatulence.
2 To slim the tummy.

THE TENSION RELEASE (PAGE 82)

This technique works on the muscles and joints in the back to relieve tension. It also strengthens the shoulders, arms, back, neck and chest.

Use specifically for the following:

1 To eliminate tension pain from between the shoulder blades and the neck.
2 To develop the chest and bust.

3 To strengthen the shoulders.
4 To slim, firm and strengthen the arms, especially the upper arms.
5 To help flatten and firm the abdominal and stomach areas.

THE CAT (PAGE 84)

This movement works on the spine, increasing both suppleness and strength. It firms the buttocks, thighs, hips and stomach and stream-lines the waist, shoulders and arms. It also strengthens the wrists, elbows and shoulders.

Use specifically for the following:

1 To eliminate backache (not caused by injury).
2 To relieve pre-menstrual tension.
3 To relieve Dysmenorrhoea.
4 To lose excess weight around the torso.
5 To trim and firm the buttocks.
6 To help eliminate digestive problems.